AROMATHERAPY

Aromatherapy is an ancient art making use of specially selected essential oils extracted from plants. Recent scientific research and modern distillation methods have enabled a therapeutic system to be built up. This book lists a selection of oils, describes the properties of each and shows how they can be used to treat a wide range of ailments.

AROMATHERAPY

The Use of Plant Essences in Healing

by

Professor Raymond Lautié
D.Sc.

with the collaboration of
André Passebecq M.D., D.Ps.

Translated from the French by
Geoffrey A. Dudley B.A.

THORSONS

THORSONS PUBLISHERS LIMITED
Wellingborough, Northamptonshire

First published 1979
Second Impression 1982

ISBN 0 7225 0394 6

Printed and bound in Great Britain by
Richard Clay (The Chaucer Press) Ltd.,
Bungay, Suffolk.

CONTENTS

                                                    Page
   Introduction   7
Chapter
1. The History of Aromatherapy   9
2. Preservation   12
3. Aromatic Essences and Their Uses   17
4. Aromatic Waters   90
5. Diseases and Aromatic Treatments   94
   Glossary   114
   Useful Address   125

INTRODUCTION

Aromatherapy consists of the use of natural aromatic essences extracted from wild or cultivated plants. These essential oils are compounds whose many organic constituents unite to produce a wide range of therapeutic and olfactory qualities.

The composition of each of them is specific, but there are small variations dependent upon the climate and soil the plant has grown in, and the methods of cultivation and distillation. The wild plant is to be preferred as it yields the most active and best balanced product, but oils extracted from cultivated plants are still good if such plants are raised sympathetically and organically. Synthetic pesticides must not be used as these are often soluble in the plants' aromatic substances; and gathering should take place at full maturity, with subsequent extraction of the oils carried out with care.

Such oils are the quintessence of plants, and they have special qualities evolved in the plant to attract insects that promote fertilization, to repel parasites, and to catalyse biochemical reactions. They can be considered to be kinds of vegetable hormones, and they have a biodynamic and ionizing potential when used therapeutically to treat human ailments. Such hyperactive extracts must be used with great care, and in suitably diluted doses, as any excess could be harmful to health simply because they are so powerful.

Complexity is the rule in biology, and every natural aroma turns out to have a quite characteristic complex association of hydrocarbons by which each constituent derives its value only from the presence of the others. In other words, each essential oil has a delicately balanced mix of basic constituents and its aromatic properties are dependent upon the molecular interplay of its component parts. Hence the need of an extraction which adequately respects these electronic links, and hence the need of suitably diluted doses which will promote and reinforce ionizations favourable to chemical processes within the body.

In the pages which follow a recommended selection of essences is examined in alphabetical order, and in each case their main therapeutic qualities are indicated.

CHAPTER ONE

THE HISTORY OF AROMATHERAPY

The origin of aromatherapy is lost in the mists of time when healers of antiquity practised their primitive natural medicine. Much later, as we learn from papyri, the Egyptian embalmers sought aromatic herbs, woods, and resins to mummify ibises, cats, monkeys, important dignitaries, and Pharaohs; arresting the putrefaction of corpses by the antiseptic power of natural essences.

Almost from the dawn of its civilization, Egypt has been famous for its botanical gardens in which were collected rare and varied plants from Africa, Arabia, and the Indies. The result was that gradually the banks of the Nile became rich in medicinal plants and renowned healing herbs to the point where they drew sages from the entire ancient world, and remedies were exchanged with Mesopotamia and Persia.

One of the founders of Pharaonic medicine was the architect Imhotep, grand vizier of King Zeser (2780-2720 B.C.), whom the people later deified. Some fourteen hundred years afterwards, a favourite of Amenhotep III (1405-1380 B.C.), who was also an architect, gave a new impulse to the art of medicine, which appeared in its full glory under the heretic sun-king Akhnaton (1370-1352 B.C.). During this period the city of Tel-el-Amarna (Akhenaton) was built according to the best rules of hygiene; in its public squares were burnt piles of aromatic substances to purify the air.

The physicians of Ionia Attica, and Crete came to improve their knowledge in the medical schools of the cities of the Nile. It was through them that there was formed the school of Cos graced by Hippocrates (460-377 B.C.), whom the Greeks in their enthusiasm named with some exaggeration the Father of Medicine. Let us not allow his successes to lead us to overlook those of his pupils or of his rivals from Turkey, Ephesus, Pergamum, or Rome – men like Celsius and Galen. The Celts also proved to be better doctors than has been taught up to now, and they enriched themselves with the knowledge of their Mediterranean colleagues.

In about the eighth century the Arabs, who were both merchants and warriors, spread the remedies from Asia Minor and the Middle East, improved the methods of extracting essential oils, perfected the apparatus for distillation, and made up new elixirs and ointments. Our own Middle Ages took inspiration from their pharmaceutical prescriptions, the science of which was taught at Grenada, Salerno, Montpellier and Paris. The great navigators of the fifteenth century, such as Bartholomew Diaz (1450-1500), Vasco da Gama (1469-1524), Christopher Columbus (1451-1506), Cortés (1485-1547), or Pizarro (1475-1541), brought back new plants and aromas from their distant voyages.

After the Renaissance, the popularity of aromatherapy waned as pharmacists developed remarkable chemical syntheses, and offered compounds which were held to be capable of replacing natural ones. At the present time this idea is gradually losing ground. It is being found that appropriately extracted and well-chosen essential oils are generally much less toxic than laboratory drugs and often even atoxic. They respect living tissues and are not subject to the disastrous habituation which calls for larger and larger doses of sulphonamides and antibiotics.

It is remarkable that the physicians of past centuries were able to discover by patient observation the main specific virtues of each aroma, which to-day we are rediscovering with the subtler means of investigation. They were able to turn them to good account in the best way; sometimes respiratory, sometimes oral, sometimes epidermal, thanks to evaporation, pulverization, or agents-solvents such as alcohol, oils, butter, and vegetable or animal fats.

More particularly, it is astonishing that they should have achieved the skill of embalming organisms by the diffusion of aromatic preparations through the skin. Let us do them the justice of acknowledging that, until the beginning of the twentieth century, our Pharmacopoeia was obliged to preserve a great deal of their aroma-based medicines.

CHAPTER TWO

PRESERVATION

The returns from the extraction of essential oils are small. They rarely exceed one per cent and sometimes drop below 0.2 per cent. Hence they are expensive products which are kept in well-stoppered flasks of coloured glass in order to prevent their deterioration by sunlight (actinic rays) and by the oxygen in the air. Moreover, it is wise to protect them from extreme variations of temperature. The best way is to keep them in glass bottles at a temperature of about 18° Centigrade (65°F).

MAIN CARRYING AGENTS

Except for rubbing on the skin or inhaling, plant essences are not used directly, but are included in solid substances or dissolved in liquids which serve them as vehicles and diluting agents. Among these are:

Water. This must be free from chlorine and without too much mineral content, but generally essential oils dissolve very little in water.

Brown sugar. In practice, three drops or so are poured on a little unrefined sugar: e.g. brown sugar or, better, whole sugar, which is much richer in calcium, phosphorus, and magnesium and for this reason is non-acidifying and anticarious.[1]

[1] This and other medical terms are defined in the Glossary (see p. 114).

Honey. As a substitute for the sugars, honey extracted by simple cold pressing from the comb is used in the same way. If possible, use honey which corresponds to the essential oil. For example, lavender essence is associated with lavender honey.

Alcohol. The ethyl alcohol derived from the distillation of wine is one of the main solvents of plant essences. Its alcoholometric strength depends on the therapeutic uses. It can vary, for instance, from 14° to 95° in spirits of aromatic herbs.

Oils. These are excellent solvents and are frequently used. Among them, I prefer those which by themselves already have an interesting therapeutic power and which are adequately resistant to rancidity. It is always necessary to use extra-pure oils obtained by first cold pressing: olive oil, peanut oil, sunflower oil, and sweet almond oil.

Vinegars. As solvents slightly superior to pure water, but much less than ethyl alcohol, wine or cider vinegars are now used quite widely in aromatherapy.

Fats. We are here concerned with solid lipids, the melting-point of which is very much higher than that of the previously-mentioned oils. Naturopaths use only non-hydrogenized vegetable fats.

Waxes. Beeswax, whitened in the sun, is most commonly used. Vegetable waxes (such as Brazilian and Montana wax) are rarely chosen because the former has a remarkable dielectric power in biodynamics.

EXTRACTION OF OILS
The main methods of extraction of essential oils are distillation, maceration, dissolving by volatile solvents, and pressing.

The most classic is open-fire distillation; the plants

and flowers are in direct contact with the water, the steam from which carries the essences into the condenser and the separator. This process calls for a great deal of care and practice to avoid the 'burning' which gives the distillate an empyreumatic smell. Water-bath or steam distillation does not have this drawback. Current preference is for vacuum distillation, which is achieved at a much lower temperature and which, consequently, respects much better the constituents of the essences, preserving them from oxidization and bad smells.

Maceration, either cold (*enfleurage*) or hot, absorbs the constituents of the plant through the intervention of vegetable oils or fats.

Dissolving with volatile solvents replaces the water of open-fire distillation with organic solvents.

Pressing is done by grating outer skins (bergamots, lemons, sweet limes, oranges) without affecting the white parenchyma. The essence runs from the torn cells into a sponge, which is then squeezed out over a container.

MAIN CONSTITUENTS

Plant essences are not readily soluble in water. At normal temperature their density lies between 0.860 (heather essence) and 1.055 (bitter almond essence), predominantly below 1.000.

Among the commonest constituents, which belong to several chemical families (alcohols, aldehydes, acids, esters, phenols, nitrogen compounds, sulphur compounds, etc.), are:

Benzyl acetate, linalyl acetate, anisic acid, myristic acid, oleic acid, benzyl alcohol, nonyl alcohol, anisic aldehyde, benzoic aldehyde, decyl aldehyde, anethole, methyl anthranilate, borneol, camphene, camphor, citral, citronellal, the esters of cinnamic acid, eucalyptol, eugenol, geraniol, hydroxycitronellal, irone, limonenes, linalol, menthol, menthone, nerol, phellandrene, pinenes, sesquiterpenes, terpenes, terpineol, vanillin, etc.

What counts first in every essential oil, what gives it its aromatherapeutic value, is not just one of the products which can be extracted from it in the purest state, but the complex *in toto*, the constituents of which are associated in particular proportions from the most important weightwise to the most diluted, right down to the oligomolecules.

Only the individualized totality possesses great biological activity, even if each of the constituents appears not to have great therapeutic qualities, which are often transformed by the rotary power of light.

In perfumery, certain essential oils are deterpenized, because too high a degree of terpenes reduces their solubility in alcohol. In aromatherapy, there is no necessity for this, and more often than not it is preferable to avoid interfering with the natural balance of the essence.

RECOMMENDED ESSENCES
Plants provide the aromatherapist with a very large number of essences, from which must be chosen the most stable in composition, the easiest to obtain, the most active for the great majority of temperaments, and the least expensive.

In this book I include only the following essential oils:

Angelica, anise, anise (Chinese), arnica, aspic, basil, bergamot, borneol, cajeput, chamomile, caraway, cardamom, carrot, centaury, cinnamon, citron, clove, coriander, cypress, elecampane, eucalyptus, fennel, garlic, gentian, geranium, ginger, goosefoot, hawthorn, heather, hyssop, juniper, laurel, lavender, ledum (wild rosemary), lemon, lime, marjoram, melissa, mints, mugwort, niaouli, nutmeg, onion, orange (Seville), origano, pine (Scots), rosemary, roses, sage, sandalwood, santolina, sassafras, savory, tangerine, tarragon, thyme (garden), thyme (wild), turmeric, turpentine, valerian, verbena, ylang-ylang.

It is by considered selection of these various essences, taken at certain hours of the day, or by special associations, that the aromatherapist succeeds in improving his patients' general condition and in overcoming their organic deficiencies. This is especially so if he adds a well-adjusted dietary regime and advises physical exercises, among which deep breathing takes first place.

In the following section each of the above essences is described, and in each case their main therapeutic properties are given.

CHAPTER THREE

AROMATIC ESSENCES AND THEIR USES

ANGELICA

(Angelica archangelica)
Fr. Angélique   Ger. Engelwurz

Active principles
Phellandrenic compounds. Organic acids. Angelicin (a coumarin). Bergaptene, imperatorin (two furanocoumarins).

Properties
Essence of angelica is colourless, but with age it first turns yellow then brown. It is used in anorexia, dyspepsia, stomach ulcers. In the form of ointments, it has a soothing effect on skin complaints, arthritis, and rheumatism. It is used in the composition of stomachics.

External uses
Arthritis: Oil-based applications (olive oil with 10% essence of angelica) or cream-based (sweet almond oil 500g + white wax 125g + tincture of benzoin 30g + essence of angelica + distilled water 350g).

Rheumatism: See Arthritis.

Skin complaints: Cover the affected parts with angelica-based cream.

Internal uses

Anorexia: Before meals, three drops of essence of angelica on a little brown sugar or in a coffee-spoonful of lavender or rosemary honey.

Stomach ulcers and dyspepsia: Between meals, three drops of essence of angelica on a little brown sugar. (Suck it very slowly.)

Expectorant: See Dyspepsia.

General restorative: For eating raw green salads at lunch, use olive oil or sunflower-seed oil with two hundred drops of essence of angelica to the litre; this corresponds per meal to less than three drops of essential oil.

ANISE

(Pimpinella anisum)
Fr. Anis vert   Ger. Anis

Active principles

Anethole. Estragole (methylchavicol). Choline. Terpenes. Resins.

Properties

Antispasmodic. Carminative. Gland stimulant. Galactogene. Diuretic. To be used with care for, in excess, essence of anise is a narcotic which slows the circulation and causes circulatory and cerebral disorders.

External uses

Applications to the thoracic cage with an essence of anise-based cream for stimulating the respiratory and circulatory organs. (Sweet almond oil 500g + white wax 125g + tincture of benzoin 30g + essence of anise 3g + distilled water 350g).

Internal uses

Asthma (bronchial spasms and coughs): Three drops on a little brown sugar, three times a day.

Colic in infants: One drop per day for each year of the child's age, with a maximum of five drops per day. Don't exceed six consecutive days.

Impotence: See Asthma.

Insufficiency of milk: Two drops on a little brown sugar or in a coffee-spoonful of lavender honey, three times a day.

Migraine and digestive dizziness: See Asthma.

Painful periods: See Asthma.

Palpitations: See Asthma.

ANISE (CHINESE STAR)

(Illicium verum)

Fr. Badiane   Ger. Sternanis

Active principles

The essence comes from the distillation of Chinese anise. It is rich in anethole, as is that from anise. Although, used in aperitifs, it is not to be recommended in home aromatherapy because of the risk of harming the nervous system if not used with care.

If need be, but in moderation, the tisane of Chinese anise (about 15g to the litre) can be used as a stomachic or carminative, once a day, after one of the main meals, or one drop of essence of Chinese anise on a little brown sugar, twice a day.

ARNICA

(Arnica montana)

Fr. Arnica   Ger. Arnika

Active principles

Flavonic heterosides. Bitters. Essential oil.

Properties

Stimulant for the circulatory system. Contusions. Ecchymoses. Vulnerary.

Internal uses
Not recommended. The oil can be dangerous and even toxic.

External uses
Tincture of arnica is employed for many different kinds of injuries; so it forms part of the family pharmacopoeia. It is prepared from 100g of dried heads which have been macerated in a litre of 90° alcohol for a fortnight. Strain and keep in a corked bottle away from the light. On using it, make the following mixture: tincture of arnica 15 ml + distilled or boiled water 45 ml + glycerine 40 ml. Apply it immediately to the area of bruising.

ASPIC

(Lavandula latifolia)
Fr. Aspic   Ger. Aspik

A variety of lavender which has the same properties as medicinal lavender but with a stronger, more camphorated smell. In aromatherapy, 30 per cent of aspic is often added to the latter to activate it.
    For uses see: LAVENDERS.

BASIL

(Ocimum basilicum)
Fr. Basilic   Ger. Basilienkraut

Active principles
Obtained by steam distillation of the leaves, the essence of the different varieties of basil is rich in estragole, linalool, lineol, ocimene, and camphor.

Properties
The plant is well-known to cooks for its fragrance, which makes it a good seasoning for raw salads and

other dishes. Like it, but more strongly so, its essence is carminative, galactogenic, stomachic, tonic. It strengthens the cortex of the suprarenal glands and the nervous system. For centuries it has been held to be antispasmodic and emmenagogic.

External uses
Insect stings: Apply to the sting one drop of essence or else oil (3 per cent sweet almond oil).

Snake bites: Allow to bleed, wash with boiled water and dab with cotton wool soaked in essence of basil. (Essence of lavender and aspic appears even more effective.)

Internal uses
The flower-heads and fresh leaves added to salads and food immediately before serving not only flavour them but also make them more digestible.

Anxiety: Three or four drops of essence on a little brown sugar or in a spoonful of lime-blossom honey, three times a day.

Gout: See Anxiety.

Insomnia: See Anxiety. If the green salad at two daily meals contains added olive or sunflower-seed oil, these drops can be replaced with three drops of essence of basil per coffee-spoonful (5 ml).

Migraine: See Insomnia.

Periods, scanty: See Anxiety.

Strain, mental: See Insomnia.

Vertigo and epilepsy: See Anxiety. Prepare a sugar compound of 100g of finely-ground brown sugar to which is added: essence of basil 1g + essence of lavender 1g + essence of rosemary 1g. From it take half a coffee-spoonful, which will serve to sweeten an infusion of verbena or mint after every meal (if one is not following a homoeopathic treatment).

BERGAMOT
(Citrus bergamia)
Fr. Bergamote   Ger. Bergamotte

Active principles
The essence is obtained by pressing the outer part of the pericarp of the fruit of the bergamot. It contains up to 50 per cent of acetate of linalyl, linalol, and dextrorotatory limonene.

Properties
As the essence is antiseptic and has a pleasant smell, it is used for intestinal colic, slow digestion, gastric spasms, and oxyures. In addition, it arouses the appetite. Lastly, it is useful for flavouring confectionery, pastries, and medicines as well as being frequently employed in the perfume industry.

External use
80° alcohol and 3-5 per cent of essence of bergamot are useful for rubbing the gastric area to combat sluggishness of the stomach.

Internal uses
Appetite, loss of: Three drops on a little brown sugar, half an hour before each meal.

Colic, intestinal: Three drops on a little brown sugar, three times a day, or use a sugar compound of 100g of powdered brown sugar with the addition of 2g of essence of bergamot + 1g of essence of lemon + 1g of essence of marjoram. From it take half a coffee-spoonful to sweeten an infusion of hot citronella after every meal.

Oxyures: Sugar compound (see Colic, intestinal).

BORNEOL OR BORNEO CAMPHOR

(Dryobalanops camphora)
Fr. Bornéol or Camphre de Bornéo

Active principles
Borneol is a natural exudation beneath the bark of the Camphora. Unlike the camphor of Japan, which is used the most, it is an *alcohol* and not a *ketone*. This fundamental difference explains its atoxicity. It should lead to only borneol being used in aromatherapy, for in the long run the other camphors are more or less toxic. Moreover, it proves much more antiseptic and even acts as a tonic, which a ketone is not. It is worth noting that hyssop and rosemary also contain borneol.

Properties
Powerful antiseptic. Cardiotonic. Antidepressive. Anti-infection.

External uses
Rheumatism: Rubbing with warm olive oil containing 10 per cent of borneol and 5 per cent of essence of chamomile or with camphorated alcohol containing the same.

Internal uses
Prepare Borneo-camphorated alcohol (10g in 100 ml of 90° alcohol scented with 3 per cent of essence of lemon). From it remove 0.5 ml (i.e. about 25 drops) and pour into a hot sweetened infusion of citronella or lemon leaves, stir, and drink rapidly (it may become cloudy). Twice a day between meals. Between five and ten years, a quarter of the full dose. Between ten and fifteen, half the dose.

This remedy disinfects the alimentary canal, strengthens the heart and the whole organism. It is to be recommended in febrile conditions and in the course of infectious illnesses.

CAJEPUT
(Melaleuca leucodendron)
Fr. Cajeput

Active principles
The essence, obtained by steam distillation of the leaves and buds of the cajeput, principally contains cineol, terpineol, pinene, and aldehydes.

Properties
Intestinal, pulmonary, and urinary antiseptic, essence of cajeput is recommended for asthma, bronchitis, dysentery, enteritis, gastric spasms, laryngitis, painful periods, and pharyngitis.

External uses
Laryngitis: Inhalation of lukewarm essence.

Neuralgia, dental: One drop of essence on the decayed tooth.

Otitis: Introduce into the ear hot olive oil with 10 per cent of Borneo camphor and 10 per cent of essence of cajeput. Plug the external auditory duct with cotton wool soaked in this oil.

Rheumatism: Rub the painful areas with the above oil.

Skin diseases: Dab the affected parts with sweet almond oil and 5 per cent of essence of cajeput.

Internal uses
Asthma: Inhale essence of cajeput. Take five drops of essence on a little brown sugar three times a day.

Bronchitis: See Asthma.

Cystitis: See Asthma.

Enteritis: See Asthma.

Gastritis (spasms): Three drops on brown sugar after each meal.

Gout: Rubbing with warm oil as described under external uses. In addition, take four drops of essence on brown sugar three times a day.

Laryngitis: See Asthma. Gargle with bicarbonated hot water (a pinch per cup and five drops of essence per 50 ml).

Oxyures: On waking and on retiring, five drops of essence on brown sugar.

Painful periods: Five drops of essence on brown sugar three times a day. Rub the lower part of the abdomen with the warm oil recommended for external uses.

Pharyngitis: See Laryngitis.

Rheumatism: See Gout.

CARAWAY

(*Carum carvi*)
Fr. Carvi   Ger. Kümmel

Active principles
The oil from ripe seeds is rich in carvone (up to 60 per cent), limonene (up to 20 per cent), carveol, dihydrocarvone, etc.

Properties
It is carminative, diuretic, galactogenic, stomachic, and vermifugal.

External uses
Dry pleurisy: Rub the thoracic cage with enriched warm oil (olive oil with 10 per cent of essence of caraway).

Rheumatism: Rub the painful areas with the above enriched oil.

Internal uses
Aerophagy: Two drops of essence on a lump of sugar after every meal.

Appetite, loss of: See Aerophagy.

Flatulence: See Aerophagy.

Lactation: Two drops of essence on sugar after each meal. Continue as necessary during breast-feeding.

Spasms, gastric: Three drops on sugar when the attack occurs. Supplement with rubbing the epigastrium with the enriched oil. (See Dry pleurisy.)

Urine, diminished amount of: See Aerophagy.

Vertigo: When the attack occurs, slowly suck some brown sugar soaked in three drops of essence.

Worms (oxyures): Three drops of essence on brown sugar between meals.

CARDAMOMS
(Elettaria cardamomum and Amomum afzelii)
Fr. Cardamomes   Ger. Kardamom

Active principles
The essences of cardamom (or cardamum) come from the distillation of either the fruit (shells and seeds) of *Elettaria cardamomum* or the white almonds of *Amomum afzelii* (grains of Paradise).

Properties
Antiseptic. Stimulative.

Internal use
Three drops of essence on brown sugar after a meal, e.g., to remove the smell of garlic and promote digestion.

CARROT, WILD

(Daucus carota)

Fr. Carotte Commune   Ger. Möhre
                          Gelbe Rübe

Active principles
The essence of wild carrot is rich in carotenes.

Properties
It is carminative and diuretic. It proves effective in dropsy, retention of urine, and digestive disorders.

Internal uses
Digestion, difficult: Three drops of essence on brown sugar after every meal.

Dropsy: Three drops between meals (morning and afternoon).

Flatulence: See Digestion, difficult.

Retention of urine: See Digestion, difficult. Supplement by rubbing the lower abdomen with warm olive oil enriched with essence of wild carrot (10 per cent).

CENTAURIES

(Erythraea centaurium, Centaurea montana, Centaurea cyanus)

Fr. Petite Centaureé
    Centaureé des Montagnes
    Centaurée Bleuet

Ger. Tausendgüldenkraut

One must distinguish the common centaury (*Erythraea centaurium*), which is a gentianaceous, the blue cornflower (*Centaurea montana*), which is a member of the compositae family, and the bluebottle (*Centaurea cyanus*), also a compositae. The two last-mentioned act rather as an infusion for bathing the eyes, preferably blue eyes, in cases of conjunctivitis. The first one, which is less bitter than gentian, contains a lactone (erythrocentaurin) and gentiopicrin as well as other active principles.

Properties

The stems, leaves, and flowers of the common centaury, which proves choleretic, febrifugal, stomachic, and tonic, are used as an alcohol infusion.

Internal uses

Digestion, slow: Four or five drops of alcohol infusion of common centaury on brown sugar.

Fevers: See Liver, sluggish.

Liver, sluggish: Allow 200g of fresh common centaury, four cloves, and a pinch of cinnamon to macerate for a week in a litre of 80° alcohol. Strain. Add a litre of boiled water. Stir well. Keep in a well-corked bottle away from the light. After each meal, suck a lump of sugar dipped in five drops of this preparation.

CHAMOMILES and MATRICARIAE

(Anthemis nobilis, matricaria chamomilla, matricaria discoidea)

Fr. Camomille Romaine
Grande Camomille
Petite Camomille

Ger. Römische Kamille
Mutterkraut
Echte Kamille

Active principles

These flowers and leaves contain essential oils, chamazulene, coumarin, heterosides, and flavonics (common chamomile); camphor, borneol, terpenes, esters, and a bitter substance (wild chamomile); and azulene (anti-allergic) (scented mayweed).

Properties

Feverfew (*Chrysanthemum parthenium*), although little used, is yet advantageous at least for its borneol and its esters. Its essence is a good counter-irritant. Perhaps its applications in homoeopathy will restore to it the place which it used to occupy in allopathy.

Wild chamomile (*Matricaria chamomilla*) had its hour of fame in the time of the Arab physicians, who used to consider it as a multivalent remedy. Its oil is hardly to be found although it has antispasmodic anti-allergic, antiphlogistic, carminative, stomachic, and vulnerary qualities. Moreover, olive oil with 10 per cent of essence of wild chamomile is highly valued in rubbing for rheumatic pains.

Alone or nearly so, common chamomile (*Anthemis nobilis*) is in general use today. It owes this popularity to the value of its infusions and essential oil. The latter, obtained by steam distillation from the flowers, is antispasmodic, antiphlogistic, anti-ophthalmic, aperitive, febrifugal, stimulative, digestive, emmenagogic, and vermifugal.

External uses

Gout and rheumatic pains: Rubbing with olive or sweet almond oil enriched with essence of chamomile (100g per litre) and of Borneo camphor (50g to 100g).

Boils, dermatitis, eczema, herpes: Dab with cotton wool soaked in the foregoing blend of oils.

Conjunctivitis: Bathing the eyes with a tisane of chamomile flowers (one soup-spoonful of flowers per cup infused for ten minutes).

Internal uses

Anaemia: Three or four drops of essence on a little brown sugar, three times a day, between meals.

Appetite, loss of: Three drops of essence on brown sugar half an hour before meals.

Congestion of the liver or spleen: See Digestion, slow. Add rubbing of the hepatic and splenic areas and spinal column with the enriched oil (see Stomach cramps).

Convulsions: See Anaemia

Depression: See Anaemia. Add rubbing of the spinal column with the enriched oil (see Stomach cramps).

Digestion, slow: After every meal, three drops of essence on brown sugar.

Fever, intermittent, in the nervous: See Digestion, slow.

Influenza: See Digestion, slow. Add rubbing of the spinal column with the enriched oil.

Insomnia: On retiring, four drops of essence on brown sugar.

Migraine: When the attack occurs, slowly suck a little brown sugar soaked in four drops of essence.

Neuralgia, facial: See Teething troubles in children.

Oxyures: Three drops of essence on brown sugar between meals. Lukewarm enema with up to 300 ml of boiled water into which a soup-spoonful of enriched olive oil has been stirred (5 drops of essence of chamomile and 5 drops of essence of garlic).

Stomach cramps: When the attack occurs, slowly suck a lump of sugar dipped in three drops of essence. Rub the epigastrium with sunflower-seed oil enriched, per litre, with 50g of borneol, 100g of essence of chamomile, 20g of essence of rosemary, and 50g of essence of sage.

Teething troubles in children: Rub the cheeks with the enriched oil (see Stomach cramps).

Vertigo: Three drops of essence on brown sugar when the attack occurs.

Baths for dermatitis: To a lukewarm bath add 300g of bicarbonate of soda (Vichy salts) enriched with essence of common chamomile (50 drops). Stir well.

N.B. Essence of *Matricaria chamomilla* or *discoidea*, also called German chamomile, has the same general indications as common chamomile. Being very bitter, it is more stimulating. Hence its use between meals. It appears especially to be more bactericidal. For this reason, it is very suitable for washing infected wounds (boiled water with the addition of 2g of essence per litre). Stir well. If necessary, filter after three days. Its effectiveness is due in particular to the azulene it contains. This solution not only avoids irritating the wounds but also strengthens the leucocytes.

CINNAMON

(Cinnamomum zeylanicum)
Fr. Cannelle de Ceylan   Ger. Zimt

Active principles
Essence of cinnamon is obtained by steam distillation from the leaves and bark of the cinnamon tree of Sri Lanka, which is more highly valued than that of China (*Laurus cassia*). It contains eugenol, cinnamic aldehyde, terpenic alcohols, benzyl benzoate, linalool, safrole, furfurol, cineol, etc.

Properties
Essence of cinnamon is antiputrescent. Antiseptic. Antidote to poison. Mildly astringent. Digestive. Haemostatic. Vermifuge.

External uses

Coughs and irritations of the respiratory organs:
Inhalations: In a litre of 90° alcohol dissolve 10g
essence of cinnamon + 30g essence of eucalyptus +
25g essence of lemon + 20g essence of lavender +
10g essence of pine + 20g essence of thyme. Pour a
soup-spoonful of the preparation into a basin of
boiling water. Reckon three inhalations per day.

Pediculosis: Rub with 30 per cent solution of
sodium sulphoricinate 100 ml + 3g essence of lemon
+ 2g essence of cinnamon + 2g essence of cloves +
2g essence of pine + 2g essence of rosemary + 2g
essence of pine.

Snake bites: Allow the bite to bleed. Wash it and
then apply a few drops of essence of cinnamon or,
better, of a mixture of equal parts of essence of
cinnamon and essence of lavender.

Internal uses

Asthenia: Three drops of essence on a little brown
sugar, three times a day outside of mealtimes.

Colic, spasmodic: See Asthenia. Supplement by
rubbing the abdomen with olive oil enriched with
essence of cinnamon (50g per litre).

Diarrhoea: See Colic, spasmodic.

Flatulence: Four drops of essence on brown sugar
after every meal.

Haemoptysis: See Flatulence. Supplement by
rubbing the thorax with olive oil enriched with
essence of cinnamon (50g per litre).

Leucorrhoea: Four drops of essence after each
meal.

Oxyures: See Leucorrhoea. 300 ml lukewarm
enema, stirring into it a soup-spoonful of olive oil
enriched with 5 drops of essence.

CITRON

(Citrus medica)

Fr. Cédrat   Ger. Zedrat

Active principles
The essence is obtained by pressing the outer skin of the fruit. Rich in terpenes, it contains a bitter principle.

Properties
Aperitive. Antiscorbutic. Restorative.

Internal uses
Appetite, loss of: Two drops of essence on a little brown sugar, half an hour before meals.

Digestion, slowness of: Stimulate the digestive secretions by taking two or three drops of essence of citron on a little brown sugar after every meal.

CLOVES

(Eugenia caryophyllata)

Fr. Girofle   Ger. (Gewürz) Nelke

Active principles
Derived by steam distillation from the flower buds of the clove tree, the essential oil contains eugenol (up to 85 per cent), aceteugenol, methyl salicylate, caryophyllene, furfurol, pinene, vanillin, etc.

Properties
Aperitive. Powerful antiseptic. Antineuralgic. Antispasmodic. Anticancer. Carminative. Stomachic. Tonic.

External uses
Dentifrice (liquid): 80° alcohol 100g + essence of anise 2g + essence of Chinese anise 2g + tincture of

benzoin 10g + essence of cloves 4g + essence of mint 8g (or, in persons who take homoeopathic remedies, essence of lemon 8g).

Lupus: Rubbing with a 10 per cent alcohol solution.

Scabies: Apply to the affected places a cream made from 1000g sweet almond oil + 250g white wax + 25g essence of cloves + 600g distilled water.

Throat and Sinusitis: Fumigations: Into boiling water pour a soup-spoonful of 80° alcohol with 8 per cent of cloves and 4 per cent essence of eucalyptus.

Vertigo: For inhalation: White wine vinegar 800 ml + 200g solid acetic acid + 50g borneol + 1g essence of cinnamon + 3g essence of cloves + 1g essence of lavender or aspic.

Wounds: Wash with distilled water and 2 per cent essence of cloves.

Internal uses
Asthenia: Three drops of essence on a little brown sugar before each meal.

Asthma: See Fumigations under Throat and Sinusitis (External uses). In addition, three drops three times a day, preferably between meals.

Childbirth (preparation for): Four drops of essence on a little brown sugar after every meal during the fortnight preceding the expected day of delivery.

Diarrhoea; Three drops of essence on a little brown sugar after every meal.

Dropsy: See Diarrhoea.

Dyspepsia: See Diarrhoea.

Flatulence: See Diarrhoea.

Gout: See Diarrhoea. In addition, rub with 80° alcohol and 10 per cent of essence of cloves.

Lungs (Asthma, Bronchitis, Pleurisy): See Asthma. Plus rubbing the thoracic cage with warm olive oil and 10 per cent of essence of cloves.

Measles: Three drops of essence on a little brown sugar three times a day.

Memory (loss of): See Asthenia.

Neuralgia, dental: See Dentifrice (External uses).

Worms (oxyures): See Asthenia. Lukewarm enema with scented water (300 ml with a soup-spoonful of olive oil and 2 per cent essence stirred into it).

CORIANDER

(Coriandrum Sativum)
Fr. Coriandre   Ger. Koriander

Active principles
Essence of coriander comes from the steam distillation of the fruit of this umbellifer, which is much prized in culinary art along with caraway, cinnamon, fennel, juniper, nutmeg, peppers, rosemary, savory, thyme, etc. In particular, it contains coriandrol (up to 80 per cent) (an isomer of borneol), cineol, borneol, geraniol, pinene, terpenes, etc.

Properties
Antispasmodic. Carminative (Flatulence). Anti-rheumatic. Digestive stimulant.

External use
Joint and rheumatic pains: Rubbing with warm olive oil and 10 per cent essence.

Internal uses
Aerophagy: 2 drops of essence on brown sugar after each meal.

Appetite, loss of: 1 drop of essence on brown sugar half an hour before each meal. For a stronger dose, 2 drops of the following blend of essences: coriander 10 ml + lemon 10 ml + caraway 10 ml + camomile 20 ml.

Digestion, slow: 2 drops of essence on brown sugar after each meal. In addition, rub the epigastrium with warm olive oil and 10 per cent essence.

Flatulence: See Aerophagy.

CYPRESS

(Cupresses sempervirens)
Fr. Cyprès   Ger. Zypresse

Active principles
The essential oil comes from distillation of the cones and contains cypress camphor, *d*-pinene, *d*-camphene, *d*-sylvestrene, cymene, sabinol, valerianic acid, etc.

Properties
Antispasmodic. Antirheumatic. Antisudorific. Astringent. Anticancer. Tonic for the veins. Nerve restorative. Vaso-constrictive.

External uses
Cicatrization of wounds: Wash with lukewarm water and 1 per cent of essential oil.

Enemas: Lukewarm water into which olive oil with 5 per cent of essence of cypress has been stirred (one soup-spoonful of oil to 300 ml of boiled water).

Internal uses

Aphonia: Three drops of essence on a little brown sugar three times a day.

Dysmenorrhoea: See Aphonia.

Haemoptysis: See Influenza.

Haemorrhoids: See Aphonia. Use the following ointment: Sweet almond oil 1000g + white wax 250g + tincture of benzoin 30g + oil of cypress 25g.

Incontinence of urine: See Aphonia. Rub the lower part of the abdomen with olive oil and 10 per cent of essential oil.

Influenza: Three drops of essence on a little brown sugar three times a day. Rub the thoracic cage with warm olive oil and 10 per cent essential oil. Inhale essence of cypress frequently.

Menopause: See Incontinence of urine.

Rheumatism: Three drops of essence on a little brown sugar after every meal. Rub the painful areas with warm olive oil and 10 per cent of essential oil.

Varicose veins: Gently apply the ointment recommended for haemorrhoids.

N.B. During a 'flu epidemic, frequently sniff essence of cypress; put several drops of it on handkerchieves and on cotton wool beside you while asleep.

ELECAMPANE

(Inula helenium)

Fr. Aunée   Ger. Echter Alant

Active principles

Essential oil containing lactones, particularly alantolactone, and the rhizome containing inulin.

Properties
The acohol preparation is bechic, cholagogic, diuretic, and tonic.

External use
To reduce itching and promote long-term healing, bathe herpes and skin eruptions with the alcohol preparation. (Let about 80g of elecampane root macerate for ten days in 30° alcohol. Strain and keep away from the light.)

Internal uses
To the above alcohol preparation add a hundred grams of honey or brown sugar per litre. When about to use, half fill a wineglass, topping it up with an equal quantity of slightly mineralized water, and drink this mixture before each of the main meals for: *Amenorrhoea, Anaemia, Bronchitis, Chlorosis, Influenza, Lack of appetite*, and *Tracheitis*.

EUCALYPTUS
(Eucalyptus globulus)
Fr. Eucalyptus   Ger. Eukalyptus

Active principles
The oil comes from the eucalyptus leaves by steam distillation. It contains eucalyptol (up to 80 per cent), aromadendrene, ethyl and amyl alcohols, butyric, caproic, and valeric aldehydes, camphene, eudesmol, phellandrene, pinene, etc.

Properties
Antiseptic (from the bactericidal point of view, the complete essence is much more active than pure eucalyptol). Soothes coughing. Antirheumatic. Febrifuge. Promotes scar formation. Vermifuge. Stimulant.

External uses

Burns and injuries: Paint with oil compound made from one litre of peanut or olive oil, 10g Borneo camphor + 4g essence of eucalyptus + 3g essence of thyme + 3g essence of lavender.

Inhalations (colds, sinusitis): To a litre of boiling water add three soup-spoonfuls of the following alcohol preparation: one litre of 90° alcohol + 30g essence of eucalyptus + 14g essence of thyme + 14g essence of pine needles + 10g essence of lemon + 10g essence of lavender.

Insects (for repelling): Use the following alcohol preparation as scent and lotion: 1 litre of 90° alcohol + 30g essence of eucalyptus + 30g essence of Ceylon grass or lemon grass (*Cymbopogon* or *Andropogon nardus*, Gramineae) + 10g essence of thyme.

Rheumatism: Rubbing of the painful areas with the following warm compound oil: one litre of olive oil + 100g camphor + 60g essential oil of eucalyptus.

Internal uses

Asthenia: Three drops of essence on a little brown sugar half an hour before each meal.

Asthma: Three drops of essence on a little brown sugar after every meal.

Bronchitis: See Asthma, Inhalations.

Colibacillosis: See Asthma. Rubbing of the abdomen (see Rheumatism).

Diabetes: See Asthma.

Influenza: See Asthma, Inhalations. Rubbing of the thoracic cage (see Rheumatism).

Laryngitis: See Asthma, Inhalations. Hot compresses on the throat with oil compound (see Rheumatism).

Measles: Three drops of essence on a little brown sugar three times a day. Inhalations (see External uses).

Rheumatism: Three drops of essence on a lump of sugar after a meal. Rubbing (see Rheumatism, External uses).

Scarlet fever: See Measles.

N.B. The sick-room gains by being disinfected by the powerful bactericide which essence of eucalyptus is. To do this, put a piece of cotton wool soaked in 80° alcohol with 40 per cent of essential oil of eucalyptus in a china dish near the patient.

FENNELS and CUMIN

Cumin, which resembles fennel, is an umbellifer with seeds like caraway. Bitter fennel and sweet fennel, too, are umbellifers. Fennel-flower or Nigella belongs to the Ranunculaceae.

Active principles
The seeds contain an essential oil from which nigellone is excluded, tannin, a bitter principle (nigelline), and a glucoside (melanthine) which is poisonous.

Properties
Antispasmodic. Carminative. Diuretic. Emmen-agogic.

Internal uses
To be used with caution. Not to be given to children under six years of age.

Bronchitis: Two drops of essence on a little brown sugar twice a day between meals.

Flatulence: Two drops of essence on a lump of sugar after each meal.

Periods, irregular: See Bronchitis.

Whooping cough (to stop the spasms): Two drops of essence on a lump of sugar during the attacks.

Worms (oxyures): Lukewarm enema (300 ml) with water into which a soup-spoonful of olive oil and 1 per cent of essence has been stirred.

GARLIC
(Allium sativum)
Fr. Ail   Ger. Knoblauch

Active principles
Allicine; sulphides; allyl sulphide and oxide; organic sulphur; organic iodine; garlicine; antibiotic allistatines I and II; nicotinamide; enzymatic allinase; various ferments; vitamins A, B_1, B_2.

Properties
Essence of garlic is a powerful intestinal and pulmonary antiseptic. Antispasmodic. Carminative. Stomachic. Cholagogic. Diuretic. Febrifuge. Anticancer. Tonic. Vermifuge. Fluidifies the blood. Cardiotonic. Hypertensive. Bactericide. Multivalent biocatalyst.

External uses
Asthenia: 100g crushed garlic in 200g of olive oil and 10g of camphor. Allow to macerate for a fortnight. Strain. Rub it into the spinal column.

Corns: Crushed-garlic plaster.

Internal uses
Arteriosclerosis: Add garlic to raw green salads. Before meals, five drops of alcohol preparation on a

little brown sugar. (Allow two hundred grams of crushed garlic to macerate in one litre of 60° alcohol. After a fortnight, strain and keep in a glass bottle away from the light.)

Asthma, Hypertension, Rheumatism: See Arteriosclerosis.

Oxyures: On waking, drink some water flavoured with garlic (one glass of the following preparation: Allow three grated cloves of garlic to macerate overnight in 100 ml of boiling water). Delicate persons prefer on waking to drink two soup-spoonsful – thirty centilitres – of syrup (infuse for one hour a litre of boiling water and 500g of crushed garlic, adding a kilo of brown sugar or honey).

GENTIAN, YELLOW
(Gentiana lutea)
Fr. Gentiane   Ger. Gelber Enzian

Active principles
The tap-root contains bitter glucosides such as gentiopicrine, gentiamarine, and amarogentine.

Properties
Bitter tonic promoting digestive secretions. Stomachic. Bile tonic. Cholagogue. The root of the yellow gentian is used in an alcohol preparation. (Crush 20g of root. Let it macerate for a day in a litre of 12°-13° white wine. Strain.) Or as a syrup. (Crush 20g of root. Let it macerate for half a day in a litre of boiled water. Strain. Add a kilo of brown sugar. Can be taken at once.)

Internal uses
Anaemia: See Fever, attacks of. Gentian increases the number of red corpuscles.

Anorexia: See Anaemia.

Diarrhoea: See Anaemia.

Digestion, slow: See Anaemia.

Fever, attacks of, and malaria: Before a meal, a small wineglassful (alchol preparation) or a liqueur-glassful (maceration).

GERANIUM (HERB ROBERT, CRANESBILL)

(Pelargonium odorantissimum or Geranium robertianum)

Fr. Géranium   Ger. Storchenschnabel

Active principles
The essential oil is obtained from the entire plant by steam distillation. It contains phenylethyl alcohol, citronellal, geraniol, linalol, terpineol, etc.

Properties
Astringent. Sedative. Insect-repellent. Antidiabetic. Anticancer. Haemostatic. Tonic. Wound-healing.

External uses
Aphthae: Rinsing the mouth with a glass of lukewarm water and a coffee-spoonful of alcohol preparation (90° alcohol and 40g of essence).

Breasts, congestion of: Bathing of the breasts with pure water (fresh if possible) and 2g of essence per litre. Or, on retiring, application of the following cream: 1000g sweet almond oil + 250g white wax + 50g essence of geranium + 600g distilled water.

Herpes: Bathing with distilled water containing 2 per cent of essential oil.

Ophthalmia: Bathing of the eyes with distilled water containing 1 per cent of essential oil.

Throat, sore: Gargling with lukewarm water. One coffee-spoonful of alcohol preparation (in accordance with the above formula) per glass of water.

Wounds: Washing with distilled water containing 2 per cent of essential oil. Application of olive oil and 10 per cent of essence. Suitable for burns.

Internal uses

Asthenia: Three drops of essence on a little brown sugar after meals.

Diabetes: See Asthenia. Rub the area of the spleen with warm olive oil and 10 per cent of essence.

Enteritis: See Asthenia. Rub the abdomen with warm olive oil and 10 per cent of essence.

Haemoptysis: See Asthenia.

Jaundice: See Asthenia.

Sterility: See Asthenia.

Tonic: See Asthenia.

Ulcer, gastric: Three drops of essence on a little brown sugar before meals. Rub the stomach with warm olive oil and 10 per cent of essence of geranium.

GINGER

(Zingiber officinale)

Fr. Gingembre   Ger. Ingwer

Active principles

The essence, which is obtained from the roots by drawing under steam, contains gingerol, gingerin, zingiberine, etc.

Properties

Antiseptic. Laxative. Febrifuge. Stomachic. Tonic.

External uses
Pains, rheumatic: Rubbing with warm olive oil and 10 per cent of essence.

Throat, sore: Gargling with boiled water which has been cooled and scented (half a coffee-spoonful of alcohol preparation and 40 per cent of essence of ginger).

Internal uses
Appetite, loss of: Three drops of essence on a little brown sugar half an hour before each meal.

Diarrhoea and intestinal disorders: See Flatulence.

Digestion, slow: See Flatulence.

Febrile conditions: Three drops of essence on brown sugar three times a day.

Flatulence: Four drops of essence on a little brown sugar after each meal.

GOOSEFOOT

(Chenopodium anthelminticum)
Fr. Chénopode or Anserine Vermifuge

Ger. Gänsefuss

Active principles
The essential oil, which is obtained by steam distillation from the flower-heads and seeds of goosefoot, contains up to 80 per cent of ascaridol, chenopodin, cymene, carvone, pure camphor, cineol, safrole, sylvestrene, volatile fatty acids, etc.

Properties
Vermifuge. This oil, which is of variable tonicity, is to be used with care. It is not to be recommended for arthritics, pregnant women, or heart, kidney, and T.B. patients.

Internal uses
Some use goosefoot oil with a great deal of caution
as a means of lowering the blood-pressure after
putting the patient on a diet high in glucides and low
in lipids. In particular, it is not to be taken on an
empty stomach.

External use
Intestinal parasites: Moist hot compresses on the
abdomen, made with infusion of goosefoot leaves.
(150g per litre. Allow to boil for ten minutes.)

N.B. Chenopodium ambrosioides or Mexican tea-
plant, a goosefoot of the composite genus Ambrosia,
is taken as a stomachic infusion. Mercury or Good
King Henry (*Chenopodium bonus henricus*) is eaten
like spinach.

HAWTHORN

(Crataegus monocya and Crataegus oxyacantha)
Fr. Aubépine   Ger. Weissdorn

For practical purposes, the different varieties have
the same medicinal properties.

Active principles
Triterpene derivatives. Flavononoids. Leuco-antho-
cyanidins. Lactone. Hyperoside. Quercetin. Vitexin.
Vitexinerhamnoside.

Properties
Notable heart tonic. Corrects arrhythmia, tachycardia, and hypertension as well as hypotension.
Combats insomnia of nervous origin. It has been
called the cardiac valerian. In addition, it acts
favourably on the capillaries.

Internal uses
Either the infusion or the tincture (200g of flowers to

the litre of 90° alcohol) can be used. Allow to macerate for a month. Strain. Keep in a corked bottle away from the light.

Angina pectoris: After the two main meals of the day, fifteen to twenty drops of the tincture in slightly mineralized water. (An attack may ensue, but this does not change the properties of the remedy.)

Arteriosclerosis: See Angina pectoris.

Cardiac weakness and fragile capillaries: See Angina pectoris.

Overwork: Ten drops of tincture dissolved in water after every meal.

Tranquillizer ('nerves'): See Overwork. At dinner the dose can be increased to twenty drops.

HEATHER
(Calluna vulgaris)
Fr. Bruyère (or Callune)   Ger. Heidekraut

Active principles
The essence is obtained by distillation from the whole plant. It contains flavonic glucosides (quercitrin and myricetrin) and arentine.

Properties
Diuretic. Antiseptic. Disorders of the urinary tracts.

Internal uses
Albuminuria: Tisane of flower-heads (30g per litre) three times a day. Three drops of essential oil on brown sugar.

Antisepsis of the urinary tracts: Three drops of essence on a little brown sugar three times a day.

Cystitis: See Antisepsis of the urinary tracts.

Lithiasis, renal: See Antisepsis of the urinary tracts.

Prostate: Mix equal parts of oil of juniper berries and essence of heather. Put four drops on a lump of sugar and take twice a day.

Rheumatism: See Antisepsis of the urinary tracts.

HYSSOP

(Hyssopus officinalis)
Fr. Hysope   Ger. Essigkraut

Active principles
Obtained by distillation of the plant, the essential oil contains borneol, geraniol, limonene, phellandrene, thujone, and slight traces of pinocamphone, which can have a certain epileptiform effect on persons predisposed. For this reason care should be taken to use it in moderation although its toxicity is inferior, for example, to that of mugwort.

Properties
Astringent. Bechic. Anticancer. Scar-forming. Digestive. Diuretic. Expectorant. Emmenagogue. Hypertensive. Sudorific. Vermifuge.

External uses
Ecchymoses: Brush on olive oil with 5 per cent of essence of hyssop.

Throat, sore: Lukewarm gargle. One coffee-spoonful of alcohol preparation (90° alcohol with 5 per cent of essence) in 100 ml of boiled water.

Wounds: Wash with distilled water and 2 per cent of essence of hyssop.

Internal uses
Appetite, loss of: Three drops of essence on a little brown sugar half an hour before each meal.

Asthma: See Throat, sore.

Atony, digestive: Three drops of essence on a little brown sugar after each meal.

Bronchitis, chronic: See Throat, sore. In addition, on retiring rub the thoracic cage with the following cream: 1000g sweet almond oil + 250g white wax + 750g distilled water + 25g essence of hyssop.

Colic: See Atony, digestive.

Coughs: See Throat, sore.

Dyspepsia: Three drops of essence on a little brown sugar before each meal.

Fevers: Three drops of essence on brown sugar three times a day. Rub the forehead with 60° alcohol containing 10 per cent borneol and 10 per cent essence of hyssop.

Flatulence: See Atony, digestive.

Gastralgia: See Atony, digestive.

Influenza: See Bronchitis, chronic.

Leucorrhoea: Three drops of essence on a little brown sugar three times a day. Rub the lower abdomen with the cream (see Bronchitis, chronic).

Lithiasis, urinary: See Leucorrhoea.

Rheumatism: Three drops of essence on a little brown sugar after each meal. Rub the afflicted part with the cream (see Bronchitis, chronic).

Throat, sore: See Throat, sore (under External uses). In addition, three drops of essence on a little brown sugar three times a day.

Worms (oxyures): Three drops of essence on a little brown sugar between meals. Lukewarm enema with scented water (300 ml into which is stirred a soup-spoonful of olive oil with 2 per cent of essence of hyssop.)

Wounds, healing of: Bathe the wounds with boiled water and 2 per cent of essence. Three times in the course of the day suck a little brown sugar soaked in three drops of essence of hyssop.

JUNIPER
(Juniperus communis)
Fr. Genévrier   Ger. Wacholder

Active principles
The essential oil is rich in alphapinene, cadinene, camphene, terpineol, terpenic alcohol, borneol, isoborneol, camphor of juniper, etc.

Properties
Antiseptic. Antirheumatic. Antidiabetic. Depurative. Diuretic. Emmenagogue. Parasiticide (external use). Carminative. Stomachic. Sudorific. Tonic.

External uses
Acne: Smear with oil and essence of juniper (olive oil with 10 per cent of essence).

Eczema, weeping: Bathe with boiled water and 2 per cent of essential oil.

Paralysis: Rubbing with oil (see Acne).

Rheumatism: See Paralysis.

Internal uses
Albuminuria: Four drops on a little brown sugar after every meal.

Arteriosclerosis: See Albuminuria.

Arthritic diathesis: See Albuminuria.

Cirrhosis: See Albuminuria. Rub the hepatic region with the blended oil (see Acne under External uses).

Cystitis: See Cirrhosis. Rub the lower abdomen with the above oil.

Diabetes: See Albuminuria. Rub the area of the spleen with the above oil.

Digestion, slow: See Albuminuria. Rub the epigastrium with the above oil.

Dropsy: Five drops of essence on a little brown sugar three times a day.

Gout: See Albuminuria. Rub the afflicted parts with the above oil.

Intestines (fermentations): Three drops of essence on a little brown sugar after every meal. Rub the abdomen with oil blended with 10 per cent of essence.

Lassitude, general: See Albuminuria.

Leucorrhoea: See Albuminuria. Rub the lower abdomen with the above oil.

Measles, scarlet fever, and other febrile ailments: See Albuminuria.

Oliguria: See Albuminuria.

Periods, painful: See Leucorrhoea.

Rheumatism: See Gout.

LAUREL

(Laurus nobilis)

Fr. Laurier   Ger. Lorbeerbaum

Active principles
From the bay laurel or sweet bay – not to be confused with the cherry laurel or common laurel

(*Prunus laurocerasus*) – are extracted essential oils. That from the berries contains cineol, geraniol, and linalool. That from the leaves is richer in cineol (up to 45 per cent) and a bitter principle.

Properties
Antirheumatic. Digestive.

External uses
Phthiriasis (skin disease caused by lice): Also known as pediculosis. Rub the infested areas with the following alcohol preparation: 1000 ml 80° alcohol + 100g camphor + 50g essence of bay laurel.

Rheumatism: Rubbing with scented olive oil and 10 per cent of essential oil of laurel or with the following cream: 1000g sweet almond oil + 250g white wax + 750g distilled water + 20g essence of laurel.

Internal uses
Digestion, slow: Three drops on a little brown sugar after each meal. One can prepare, as a digestive, an infusion of (preferably fresh) laurel leaves – two or three to the cup; add sugar and one drop of essence of laurel.

LAVENDERS
(Lavandula officinalis)
Fr. Lavandes   Ger. Lavendel

Active principles
Aromatherapy makes use of different varieties of lavender, all equally active but differing somewhat in their perfume. Among them are worth mentioning *Lavandula spica stoechas* with a more penetrating smell and better for respiratory complaints; spike lavender or French lavender (*Lavandula spica latifolia*) with a more camphorated smell; and, finally, *Lavandula officinalis* with a more delicate

perfume and also the most widely used.

Obtained by dry steam distillation from the flower-heads, the essence is rich in d-borneol, caryophyllene, cineol, coumarin, geraniol, limonene, linalol, l-pinene, esters of geranyl, linalyl, butyric acid, and valerianic acid. The composition depends to a great extent on the type of lavender, its culture, the local microclimate, and the year. (Two hundred kilos of flowers yield from 750g to 1000g of essence.)

Properties

Analgesic. Antimigraine. Antirheumatism. Antiseptic. Antispasmodic. Bechic. Sedative for the nerves of the heart. Cholagogue. Heals wounds. Diuretic. Aids digestion by increasing the secretions of the alimentary canal. Lowers blood-pressure. Insecticide. Parasiticide. Sudorific. Heart tonic.

External uses

Acne: Bathe with lavender-water (distilled water with 2 per cent of essence); then apply lavender-cream (1000g sweet almond oil + 250g white wax + 750g distilled water + 20g essence of lavender + 5g aspic). Some favour the direct treatment with lavender alcohol (1000g 80° alcohol + 60g essence of lavender).

Burns: Paint with lavender oil (1000g olive oil + 100g essence of lavender).

Inhalations (for asthmatics and sufferers from sinusitis): Pour into distilled water (100 ml) a coffee-spoonful of 60 ml essence of lavender + 20 ml essence of pine + 40g essence of eucalyptus + 20 ml essence of thyme.

Insects: Essence of lavender applied direct to the stings.

Leucorrhoea: Vaginal douches of lukewarm water with 2 per cent of essence of lavender.

Pediculosis: Rub with 80° alcohol and 40 per cent of essence of lavender.

Snake bites: Allow the bite to bleed, then dab with pure essence of lavender or, better still, with a mixture of 60 ml lavender + 40 ml aspic.

Wounds: Wash with distilled water and 2 per cent of essence. Brush with olive oil and 10 per cent of essence.

Internal uses

Asthma: Inhalations (see Inhalations under External uses). In addition, between meals, three or four drops of essence on a little brown sugar.

Chlorosis: Four drops of essence on a little brown sugar half an hour before each meal.

Coughs: See Chlorosis. Gargling with lukewarm lavender-water. (To 100 ml of boiled water add one coffee-spoonful of: 1000 ml 80° alcohol + 20 ml essence of eucalyptus + 60 ml essence of lavender.)

Cystitis: See Chlorosis. In addition, rub the lower abdomen with the lavender-cream (see Acne).

Digestion, slow: Four drops of essence on a little brown sugar after each meal. Rub the epigastrium with 80° alcohol and 40 per cent of essence of lavender.

Enteritis: Four drops of essence on a lump of sugar three times a day. Rub the abdomen with lavender-cream (see Acne) or 10 per cent lavender-oil.

Heart, nervous: See Chlorosis. Rub the heart region with lavender oil and 10 per cent of essence.

Hysteria: See Chlorosis.

Infectious diseases: See Chlorosis. Rub the body with lavender alcohol and 40 per cent of essence.

Leucorrhoea: See Leucorrhoea (External uses). In addition, three drops of essence on a little brown sugar after each meal.

Measles: See Chlorosis. Add the inhalations (see Inhalations under External uses).

Migraine: Three drops of essence on a little brown sugar after each meal. Fresh compresses on the forehead and nape of the neck with the following alcohol preparation: 1000 ml 80° alcohol + 100g Borneo camphor + 40 ml essence of lavender + 20 ml essence of aspic.

Neurasthenia: See Chlorosis. Rub the spinal column with the above alcohol preparation.

Paralysis: See Chlorosis. Rub the spinal column and the paralysed part with the following alcohol preparation: 1000ml 80° alcohol + 40 ml essence of lavender + 20 ml essence of aspic + 30 ml essence of basil.

Periods, scanty: Four drops of essence three times a day. Rub the lower abdomen with the following: 1000ml olive oil + 100g camphor + 60g essence of lavender. Some people prefer to rub with the above alcohol preparation.

Spasms: See Chlorosis.

Worms (oxyures): After every meal, four drops of essence on a little brown sugar. Lukewarm lavender enema (300 ml of boiled water into which a soup-spoonful of olive oil with 10 per cent of essence of lavender has been stirred.)

LEDUM (WILD ROSEMARY)

(Ledum palustre)

Fr. Romarin Sauvage or Lédon   Ger. Sumpfforst

Active principles

The entire plant contains an essential oil rich in a camphor – ledol – arbutin and leditannic acid. Sometimes used as an abortifacient and, in weak doses, as a diuretic, it requires discernment in its internal use for it quickly irritates the digestive organs and the nerves, especially on account of the toxicity of ledol. It is better to use it externally only.

External uses

Pediculosis: In formulas for products based on essence of rosemary, the latter can be partly replaced (up to 30 per cent) by essence of marsh ledum.

Scabies: See Pediculosis.

LEMON

(Citrus limonum)

Fr. Citronnier   Ger. Zitrone

Active principles

The essence is extracted by pressing the outer portion of the pericarp. (The green fruits are richer in it than the ripe ones.) To obtain one kilo, more than three thousand lemons are needed. It contains terpenes (camphene, limonene, phellandrene, pinene, sesquiterpenes), citral, citronellal, linalool, acetates of linalyl and geranyl, aldehydes, camphor of lemon, etc.

Properties

Powerful non-toxic bactericide. Alkali-forming. Sedative. Regulator of stomach acidity. Hypotensive.

Carminative. Laxative. Heart tonic. Diuretic. Antirheumatic. Stimulates the white corpuscles. Haemostatic.

External uses

Herpes: Dab with cotton wool soaked in water with 2 per cent of essence of lemon.

Insect bites and stings: One drop of essence on the bite or sting.

Nails, brittle: Every evening, immerse them for a quarter of an hour in warm olive oil with 10 per cent of essence of lemon. Do the same for chilblains.

Otitis: Into the auditory duct pour a little lukewarm sweet almond oil with 10 per cent of essence of lemon.

Scabies: Brush with 60° alcohol and 20 per cent of essence of lemon.

Throat, sore: Gargling with lukewarm boiled water and 2 per cent essence of lemon.

Thrush: Rinsing the mouth with the above solution or with lemonade (dilute the pure juice with the same volume of water) enriched with 10 drops of essence per 100 ml. Stir well.

Verrucae: Dab them each evening with essence of lemon.

Warts: See Verrucae.

Wound: Bathe with boiled water and 2 per cent of essence of lemon. Arrests the flow of blood.

Wrinkles, facial: On retiring, nourish the skin with the following cold cream: 1000g sweet almond oil; 250g white wax; 30g tincture of benzoin; 750g distilled water; 20g essence of lemon.

Internal uses

Aerophagy: Five drops of essence on a little brown sugar after meals.

Ageing: Four drops of essence of lemon on brown sugar after every meal. Massage of the spinal column, thorax, and abdomen with lemon water (80° alcohol with 30g of essence of lemon).

Anaemia: Five drops of essence on brown sugar half an hour before meals.

Appetite, loss of: See Anaemia.

Arteriosclerosis: Five drops on brown sugar three or four times a day.

Asthenia: See Anaemia. In addition, once a day rub the spinal column with olive oil and 10 per cent of essence of lemon.

Blood, hyperviscosity of: See Liver complaints.

Calcium, loss of: See Aerophagy.

Capillaries, fragile: See Aerophagy.

Convalescence: See Asthenia.

Dysentery: See Aerophagy. In addition, rub the abdomen with warm olive oil and 10 per cent of essence.

Growth: See Asthenia.

Hypertension: Three drops of essence on brown sugar after every meal. In addition, once a day rub the region of the heart with warm olive oil and 10 per cent essence of lemon.

Infectious diseases: Three drops of essence on brown sugar four times a day.

Influenza: See Asthenia.

Jaundice: See Liver complaints.

Lithiasis, biliary: See Liver complaints. In addition, rub the area of the liver once or twice a day with warm olive oil and 10 per cent of essence of lemon.

Liver complaints: Three drops of essence on brown sugar after every meal.

Lungs (asthma, bronchitis, pleurisy): Five drops of essence on brown sugar three times a day. From time to time inhale essence of lemon. Once a day massage the thorax and the spinal column with warm olive oil and 10 per cent of essence of lemon.

Malaria: Five drops of essence on brown sugar four times a day.

Rheumatism: Three drops on a lump of sugar after every meal. Rub the painful areas with warm olive oil and 10 per cent of essence or with the cold cream indicated under Wrinkles, facial.

Stomach, hyperacid: See Liver complaints. In addition, rub the epigastrium with warm olive oil and 10 per cent of essence.

N.B. Infusions of lemon leaves and flowers, sweetened with honey or brown sugar, are strengthened by adding to them one drop of essence of lemon per 10 ml.

Lemon baths are noteworthy for invigorating the skin. (For each bath, dissolve 350g of sodium bicarbonate enriched with 20g of essence of lemon or add a tisane of lemon leaves – 200g in two litres of water. The boiled leaves are added in a strainer.)

LIME BLOSSOM

(*Tilia cordata* – Small-leaved lime. *Tilia platyphyllos* – Broad-leaved lime.)

Fr. Tilleul   Ger. Kleinblätterige Linde (Small-leaved lime).

Sommerlinde (Broad-leaved lime).

Active principles
The flowers of the two varieties of lime contain identical essential oils, which are given a pleasant fragrance by farnesol.

Common properties
Antispasmodic. Bechic. Diaphoretic. Emollient.

Internal uses
Liver pains: Three drops of essence on a little brown sugar during the attack.

Lungs (Bronchitis, Pleurisy): Four drops of essence on a little brown sugar after every meal.

Spasms, digestive: Slowly suck a little brown sugar steeped in three drops of essence.

Stomach cramps: See Liver pains.

MARJORAM, SWEET

(Origanum marjorana)
Fr. Marjolaine   Ger. Wurstkraut

Not to be confused with *Origanum vulgare* (Common marjoram) and other origans considered later.

Active principles
All parts of the cultivated marjoram contain an essential oil which is extracted by steam distillation and which includes camphor, borneol, terpenes (origanol, pinene, sabinene, terpineol), etc.

Properties
Antispasmodic. Carminative. Digestive. Expectorant. Hypertensive. Vasodilator. Vulnerary. It must be used with moderation so as not to blunt the feelings and thus produce in some patients a certain deadening effect.

External uses
For invigorating baths, add to the water a few soup-spoonsful of the following alcohol preparation: 1000 ml 90° alcohol + 40g essence of lemon + 60 ml essence of lavender + 30 ml essence of thyme.

Internal uses
Aerophagy: Four drops of essence on a little brown sugar after each meal.

Anxiety: See Aerophagy.

Blood-pressure: Sweet marjoram being an arterial vasodilator, take five drops of essence on a lump of sugar between meals.

Bronchitis: Three drops of essence on a little brown sugar three times a day. From time to time inhale the pure essence.

Digestion, slow: See Aerophagy.

Insomnia: Three drops of essence on a little brown sugar half an hour before retiring.

Migraine: See Aerophagy. Rub the temples, forehead, and nape of the neck with marjoram alcohol (1000 ml 80° alcohol + 100g borneol + 60g essence of sweet marjoram).

Neurasthenia: See Aerophagy. Rub the spinal column with the above alcohol.

Wounds: Wash with distilled water and 2 per cent essence.

MELISSA (BALM)

(Melissa officinalis)
Fr. Mélisse   Ger. Zitronenkraut

Active principles
The essential oil contains linanol, geraniol, citronellal, citral, aldehydes, etc.

Properties
Antispasmodic. Carminative. Diaphoretic. Sedative. Stomachic.

Internal uses
Aerophagy: Three drops of essence of melissa on a little brown sugar after every meal.

Colic: see Aerophagy.

Flatulence: See Aerophagy.

Spasms, gastric: See Aerophagy. A tisane of melissa flower-heads, cloves (two per cup), and a little cinnamon soothes stomach pains.

Stomach cramps: See Aerophagy.

MUGWORT

(Artemisia absinthum and *Artemisia vulgaris)*
Fr. Absinthe, Armoise   Ger. Geissfuss

Active principles
Cineol and bitter principle.

Properties
Choleretic and vermifuge. Laxative. Regulates the female cycle. Digestive. Often employed by liqueur distillers.

External uses
Wounds, suppurating: Cleanse them with boiled water into which has been poured half a coffee-spoonful of a preparation of 30g of essence to the litre of 90° alcohol.

Internal uses
Do not use this essence systematically and continuously as it may lead to intestinal and nervous disorders. Not recommended during pregnancy and breast-feeding.

Aperitif: Three drops of essence on a little brown sugar just before lunch.

Atony, gastric: Three drops after every meal for six days, then stop for a week, and so on.

Diuretic: See Aperitif.

Emmenagogue: See Atony, gastric.

Febrifuge: See Atony, gastric.

Oxyures: Over six and under ten years of age, three drops in a coffee-spoonful of lavender honey once a day (twice a day between ten and fifteen years).

NIAOULI
(Melaleuca viridiflora)

Active principles
Essence of niaouli, sometimes called gomenol, comes from the distillation of the leaves of the Melaleuca. In the same family is found *Melaleuca cajuputi* or *Melaleuca leucodendron*, from which is extracted essence of cajeput. The main constituents of the essential oil of niaouli are eucalyptol, terpineol, citrene, laevorotatory limonene, dextro-rotatory pinene, terebenthene, acetic, butyric, valerianic esters, etc.

Properties
Anticatarrhal. Antirheumatic. Balsamic. Tissue stimulant. Vermifuge.

External uses
Bronchitis: Inhale the following preparation: 1000 ml 80° alcohol + 10 ml essence of eucalyptus + 40 ml essence of lavender + 50 ml essence of niaouli. And rub the chest with it.

Epidemics: At the time of an epidemic, put a few

drops of the following on a handkerchief: 1000 ml 90° alcohol + 10g essence of mint + 30g essence of eucalyptus + 60g essence of lavender + 60g essence of niaouli. Inhale it frequently.

Throat: Lukewarm gargle (100 ml boiled water + one half-coffee-spoonful of 1000 ml 80° alcohol + 20 ml essence of eucalyptus + 60 ml essence of niaouli.)

Ulcers: Wash with aromatic distilled water and 2 per cent of essence of niaouli. Brush with aromatic oil (100 ml olive oil + 5 ml essence of lemon + 15 ml essence of niaouli). Suitable also for burns.

Wounds: See Ulcers.

Internal uses
Bronchitis: See under External uses. Slowly suck a little brown sugar impregnated with three drops of essence.

Enteritis: Three drops of essence on a little brown sugar after each meal. Rub the abdomen with the alcohol preparation recommended for Epidemics (External uses).

Infections, puerperal: See Enteritis.

Infections, urinary: See Enteritis.

NUTMEG
(Myristica fragrans)
Fr. Noix Muscade　　　Ger. Muskatnuss

Active principles
Obtained by steam distillation from the fruit of the nutmeg-tree, the essential oil contains *d*-camphene, dipentene, *d*-pinene, borneol, geraniol, linalool, terpineol, eugenol, safrole, myristicin, etc.

Properties
Carminative. Dissolves biliary calculi. Digestive.

Stimulant. Avoid large doses, which bring on nervous and mental disorders.

External use
Rheumatism: Rubbing with aromatized oil (olive oil with 10 per cent of essence).

Internal uses
Asthenia: Two drops of essence on a little brown sugar after each meal.

Diarrhoea: See Asthenia. In addition, rubbing of the abdomen with the aromatized oil (see Rheumatism under External use).

Digestion, slow: See Asthenia.

Flatulence: See Asthenia.

Gastralgia: See Asthenia. Rubbing of the epigastrium with the above-mentioned aromatized oil.

Lithiasis, biliary: Two drops of essence on a little brown sugar after each meal. Rubbing of the area of the liver with the above-mentioned aromatized oil.

ONION

(Allium cepa)
Fr. Oignon   Ger. Zwiebel

Active principles
This bulb, which has been known from very ancient times, yields an essence rich in allylpropyl disulphide, flavones, etc.

Properties
Bacteriostatic. Disinfectant. Antirheumatic. Anti-infection better than pharmaceutical antibiotics. Antisclerous. Antiscrofula. Lowers blood-sugar level. Diuretic. Antiureal. Expectorant. Digestive.

External uses

Abscesses: Bathe with the water in which an onion has been cooked. Prepare the following: Allow 500g of chopped onions to macerate for a fortnight in 500g of 60° alcohol. Strain and use for bathing the abscesses.

Boils: See Abscesses.

Stings: Dab with the onion alcohol preparation (see Abscesses).

Worms: Lukewarm enema with water in which an onion has cooked.

Wounds: See Abscesses.

Internal uses

In everything that follows, raw onion is a choice food that can back up the alcohol preparation.

Aging, Arteriosclerosis, Arthritic diathesis, Asthenia, Asthma, Atony (digestive), Azotaemia, Bronchitis, Colds, Diabetes, Diarrhoea, Flatulence, Growth, Imbalance (glandular), Impotence, Lithiasis (biliary), Lymphatism, Obesity, Oedemas, Oliguria, Pericarditis, Pleurisy, Prostate gland (enlargement of), Rheumatism, Rickets, Strain (mental and physical), and *Worms* are not only all the better for daily consumption of raw onion, but are also more effectively seen to by a soup-spoonful of the alcohol preparation (see Abscesses) taken at the *start* of every meal. (Its taste can be improved by sugar and lemon juice.)

ORANGE, SEVILLE

(Citrus vulgaris or Citrus bigaradia)
Fr. Bigaradier or Oranger Amer   Ger. Pomeranze

Active Principles

Obtained by steam distillation from the fresh blossom, essence of orange flowers contains geraniol, linanol (up to 30 per cent), nerol, indol, jasmone, anthranilic, benzoic, phenylacetic esters, etc. (essence of neroli).

Properties
Sedative. Mildly hypnotic.

Internal uses
Diarrhoea, chronic: Three drops of essence on a little brown sugar after each meal.

Insomnia: Three drops of essence on a little brown sugar or in an infusion (sweetened with sugar or honey) of orange or lemon leaves just before retiring.

Palpitations: Three drops of essence on a little brown sugar three times a day.

ORIGAN(UM)(WILD MARJORAM)
(Origanum vulgare, Origanum floribundum, and Origanum glandulosum)
Fr. Origan   Ger. Wilder Majoran

Often known as common marjoram or wild marjoram.

Active principles
The essential oil of origan contains thymol (up to 16 per cent), carvacrol, origanene, etc.

Properties
Laxative. Antispasmodic. Carminative. Antiseptic. Bechic. Expectorant. Diaphoretic. Emmenagogue. Parasiticide. Stomachic. Tonic.

External uses
Cellulitis: Rubbing with origan cream: 1000g sweet almond oil + 250g white wax + 750 ml distilled (or

rose-) water + 50g tincture of benzoin + 20g essence of origan.

Pediculosis: Rubbing with the following preparation: 1000 ml 80° alcohol + 20g essence of thyme + 20g essence of geranium + 50g essence of origan.

Rheumatism: Rubbing either with the following preparation: 1000 ml 80° alcohol + 20g essence of rosemary + 50g essence of origan (or with origan oil) 1000 ml olive oil + 50g essence of origan.

Internal uses

Aerophagy: Three drops of essence on a little brown sugar after each meal.

Appetite, loss of: Three or four drops of essence on a little brown sugar half an hour before each meal.

Asthma: See Aerophagy.

Bronchitis: See Aerophagy.

Coughs: Four drops of essence on a little brown sugar just as the fits of coughing come on.

Digestion, slow: See Aerophagy.

Periods, scanty: Four drops of essence on a little brown sugar between meals.

Rheumatism: See Aerophagy. In addition, rubbing (see Rheumatism under External uses).

PEPPERMINT

(Mentha piperita)

Fr. Menthe poivrée   Ger. Pfefferminze

Different mints are known, of which the one most used is peppermint. However, we should not overlook Corsican mint *(Mentha requienii)*, pennyroyal (*Mentha pulegium*), spearmint (*Mentha spicata*).

Active principles
Obtained by steam distillation from the leaves and flower-heads, the essences of mint are of a fairly variable composition according to the species and the climate. They are more active in cold regions; hence the success of the Mitcham variety. Found in them are menthol, menthone, limonene, menthene, phellandrene, etc.

Properties
Antilactation. Anti-insect. Antiseptic. Antispasmodic. Carminative. Emmenagogue. Stimulant. Stomachic. Parasiticide. Vermifuge. It should not be used unduly for it may result in irritating the stomach and disturbing sleep on account of high doses of menthol, especially in certain people.

External uses
Asthma: Inhalations. (Into 100 ml of boiled water pour a coffee-spoonful of mentholated alcohol – 1000 ml 80° alcohol + 60 ml essence of mint fortified, if necessary, with 40 ml essence of eucalyptus.)

Bronchitis: See Asthma.

Migraine: Inhale essence of mint. (For inhalations see Asthma.)

Mosquito repellent: To repel mosquitoes, put a few drops of essence on the sheets.

Mouthwash: Use the following: 1000 ml 90° alcohol + 40 ml essence of mint + 10 ml essence of Chinese anise + 10 ml essence of anise + 4 ml essence of cloves + 2 ml essence of cinnamon. Put half a coffee-spoonful of this in a glass of water for rinsing the mouth and also for gargling.

Scabies: Apply the following cream to the affected parts: 1000g sweet almond oil + 250g white wax + 750g distilled water + 30g essence of mint.

Sinusitis: See Migraine.

Internal uses

Aerophagy: Four drops of essence of mint on a little brown sugar after every meal.

Asthma: See Asthma (External uses). In addition, five drops of essence of mint on a little brown sugar between meals.

Atony, digestive: Three drops of essence of mint after every meal.

Bronchitis, chronic: See Asthma.

Colic: Four drops of essence on a little brown sugar three times a day.

Flatulence: See Atony, digestive.

Food poisoning: See Atony, digestive.

Indigestion: See Atony, digestive.

Liver ailments: See Atony, digestive. Rubbing of the liver area with the above-mentioned cream.

Migraine: Five drops of essence on a little brown sugar. Mentholated-alcohol compresses (1000g alcohol + 5g camphor + 20g essence of mint).

Palpitations: See Atony, digestive.

Paralysis: Five drops of essence on a little brown sugar after every meal. Rub the paralysed area with the mentholated cream (see Scabies under External uses).

Worms (oxyures): Five drops of essence on a little brown sugar outside of mealtimes, particularly on retiring.

PINE, SCOTS

(Pinus sylvestris)

Fr. Pin sylvestre   Ger. Waldkieferföhre

Active principles

Well known is the oil from the buds (wrongly called fir buds), the oil from resin (or turpentine), and the oil from pine needles. They are all rich in aromatic compounds. Turpentine will be examined later. Only the oil from needles is considered here. It contains bornyl acetate, cadinene, pumilone, pinene, sylvestrene, carene, limonene, etc.

Properties

Respiratory-tract antiseptic. Liver antiseptic. Urinary antiseptic. Revitaliser. Antirheumatic.

External uses

Bronchitis: Inhalations. (Pour one coffee-spoonful of the following preparation into 100 ml of boiling water: 1000 ml 90° alcohol + 15g pine-needle oil; or else 1000 ml 90° alcohol + 25g essence of eucalyptus + 10g essence of thyme + 5g essence of lavender + 15g pine-needle oil.) Rub the thoracic cage with olive oil plus 5 per cent of pine-needle oil.

Rheumatism: Rub with the above alcohol preparation or with the following cream: 1000 ml sweet almond oil + 250g white wax + 750g distilled water + 20g essential oil of pine.

Internal uses

Asthma: Five or six drops of essential oil on a little brown sugar after each meal.

Bronchitis: See Asthma; also Bronchitis under External uses.

Colic: See Asthma. Rub the abdomen with the cream indicated for Rheumatism.

Cystitis: See Asthma.

Influenza: See Bronchitis.

Lithiasis, biliary: Four drops of essential oil on a little brown sugar after each meal.

Pneumonia: See Bronchitis.

Prostatitis: Six drops of essential oil on a little brown sugar after each meal.

Rickets: See Prostatitis. Rub the spinal column with the alcohol preparation recommended for Bronchitis under External uses.

Stomach cramps: When the pain attacks, five drops of essential oil on a little brown sugar. Can be repeated four times a day.

N.B. During a period of epidemic, put by the bedside a saucer containing some conifer resin cut into small pieces + 10 per cent essence of turpentine + 5 per cent alcohol preparation recommended for Bronchitis under External uses.

ROSE, FRENCH
(Rosa gallica)
Fr. Rose   Ger. Essigrose

Active principles
The essential oil of the red or Provence rose is very expensive, so that it is not much used in aromatherapy. It is most frequently replaced by rose-water, which is much cheaper.

External uses
Hardening of the skin: Wash with rose vinegar, well diluted with water. Or else with vinegar and 0.5 per cent of rose essence, again diluted to suit.

Throat, inflamed and sore: Astringent gargle with an infusion of 40 per cent of petals. Eat rose honey. (Let 80g to 100g of petals infuse for a day in 100g of boiling water. Strain. Add 100g of honey. Allow to simmer over a low flame until the consistency is that of a thick syrup.) One can also gargle with rose vinegar derived from the ten-day maceration of 100g of dried, well-chopped petals in a good wine vinegar (lukewarm gargling with two coffee-spoonsful to a glass of water).

Internal uses
Diarrhoea: Infusion of petals (60g per litre) between meals.

ROSEMARY

(Rosmarinus officinalis)
Fr. Romarin   Ger. Rosmarin

Active principles
The essential oil contains borneols (up to 15 per cent), camphene, camphors, cineol, lineol, pinene, resins, a bitter principle, saponin, etc.

Properties
Antidiarrhoea. Antifermentescible. Antirheumatic. Antineuralgic. Cardiotonic. Carminative. Bechic. Diuretic. Sudorific. Cholagogue. Hypertensive. Parasiticide. The very potent essential oil of rosemary must be taken in moderation. Any excess incurs the risk of bringing on epileptiform seizures and poisoning.

External uses
Burns: Wash with boiled water and 2 per cent of essence. Paint with perfumed olive oil (1000 ml olive oil + 60g essence of rosemary).

Pediculosis: Smear the affected parts with 100 ml

olive oil + 5 ml essence of cinamon + 10 ml essence
of rosemary.

Rheumatism: Hot compresses soaked in boiled
water with 2 per cent of essence. For pain rub with
90° alcohol and 6 per cent of essence or, better, with
perfumed olive oil (see Pediculosis). Scented
morning baths – pour in one or two soup-spoonsful
of alcohol preparation (80° alcohol with 6 per cent of
essence).

Scabies: See Pediculosis.

Wounds: See Burns.

Internal uses
Asthma: Three drops of essence on a little brown
sugar after each meal.

Bronchitis, chronic: See Asthma. Rub the spinal
column with perfumed olive oil (see Burns under
External uses).

Chlorosis: Four drops of essence on a little brown
sugar, half an hour before each meal.

Cholecystitis: Four drops of essence on a little
brown sugar after each meal. Rub the area of the
liver with perfumed olive oil (see Burns under
External uses).

Cirrhosis: See Cholecystitis.

Colic: Five drops of essence on a little brown sugar
after meals. Rub the abdomen with 60° alcohol and 3
per cent of essence of rosemary.

Debility, general: Four drops of essence on a little
brown sugar before each meal. Rub the spinal
column with 60° alcohol and 3 per cent of essence of
rosemary or, better still, with the following cream:
1000 ml sweet almond oil + 250g white wax + 750g
distilled water + 25g essence of rosemary.

Diarrhoea: See Colic.

Digestion, slow: See Colic.

Dizzy spells: See Fainting spells.

Dysmenorrhoea: See Leucorrhoea.

Fainting spells: When the indisposition occurs, slowly suck a little brown sugar steeped in six drops of essence. This can be repeated four or five times a day.

Flatulence: Four or five drops of essence on a little brown sugar after each meal.

Heart trouble (of nervous origin): See Flatulence.

Hypercholesterolaemia: See Flatulence.

Leucorrhoea: See Flatulence.

Lithiasis, biliary: See Cholecystitis.

Liver ailments: See Cholecystitis.

Lymphatism: See Debility, general.

Migraine: See Flatulence.

Rheumatism: Five drops of essence on a little brown sugar before each meal. In addition, rubbing (see Rheumatism under External uses).

SAGE

(Salvia officinalis)
Fr. Sauges   Ger. Salbei

There are other sages besides the one above: meadow sage (*Salvia pratensis*); whorled sage (*Salvia verticillata*); and clary (*Salvia sclarea*). They all yield essential oils of closely related composition. Some, however, can be more or less toxic, even in moderate doses, for some people. So, to be safer, oil of clary, which is non-toxic, is generally used.

Active principles
Essence of herb sage contains thujone (up to 45 per cent), borneol, sage camphor (salviol), cineol, salvene, salvone, etc. Essence of clary is rich in sclareol.

Properties
Antiseptic. Antispasmodic. Antisudorific. Laxative. Astringent. Scar-forming. Depurative. Diuretic. Emmenagogic. Stabilizes the vagosympathetic system. Hypertensive. Stimulant. Stomachic. Tonic.

External uses
Alopecia: Rub with 40° alcohol and 3 per cent of essence of herb sage.

Aphthae: Rinse the mouth with distilled water and 2 per cent of essence of herb sage.

Asthma: Gargling (pour into 100 ml of boiled water half a coffee-spoonful of 80° alcohol with 6 per cent of essence of herb sage).

Eczema: Bathe with distilled water and 2 per cent of essence; then paint with olive oil and 10 per cent of essence.

Insect bites and stings: One drop of essence applied to the sting.

Laryngitis: Lukewarm gargling with distilled water and 2 per cent of essence.

Leucorrhoea: Douche of boiled water with 2 per cent of essence of herb sage.

Throat, sore: See Asthma.

Ulcers: Compresses with boiled water and 2 per cent of essence. Apply the following cream: 1000 ml olive or peanut oil + 250g white wax + 750 ml distilled water + 25g essence of sage.

Wounds: Cleanse with boiled water and 2 per cent of essence. Apply the cream as for Ulcers.

Internal uses (use clary)

Adenitis: Two drops of essence on a little brown sugar after each meal.

Apoplexy: See Adenitis.

Asthma: See Asthma under External uses. In addition, three drops of essence of clary on a little brown sugar after each meal.

Bronchitis, chronic: See Asthma.

Convalescence: See Exhaustion, mental and physical.

Diarrhoea: See Adenitis.

Digestion, slow: See Diuresis, inadequate.

Diuresis, inadequate: Three drops of essence of clary on a little brown sugar after each meal.

Exhaustion, mental and physical: Three drops of essence of sage on a little brown sugar half an hour before every meal.

Fever, intermittent: See Diuresis, inadequate.

Hypotension: See Diuresis, inadequate.

Lymphatism: See Exhaustion, mental and physical.

Menopause: See Diuresis, inadequate.

Milk secretion (to stop): See Diuresis, inadequate. The use of sage dries up the secretion.

Neurasthenia: See Diuresis, inadequate.

Night-sweats and sweaty hands: See Diuresis, inadequate.

Periods, scanty: See Diuresis, inadequate.

Vertigo: When the attack occurs, slowly suck a little brown sugar steeped in three drops of essence of clary. Repeat three times in the course of the day.

SANDALWOOD

(Santalum album and *Santalum spicatum)*
Fr. Santal   Ger. Sandelholz

Active principles
By steam distillation sandalwood yields an essential oil rich in various terpenic alcohols, including fusanols and santalol, in various santalic and teresantalic alcohols, and in hydrocarbons.

Properties
Astringent. Pulmonary antiseptic. Urinary antiseptic. Tonic.

External uses
Powdered sandalwood, impregnated with sandal-wood oil, burns giving off a pleasant smell and antiseptic vapours (a procedure formerly used in religious ceremonies). In a saucer by the bedside in sick-rooms put some cotton wool soaked in sandalwood essence.

SANTOLINA (LAVENDER COTTON)

(Santolina chamaecyparissus)
Fr. Santoline or Petit Cyprès

Active principles
Its essential oil is extracted from the seeds.

Properties
Antispasmodic. Emmenagogue. Stimulant. Vermi-fuge.

Internal uses
Emmenagogue: Five drops on a little brown sugar

after each meal. Take immediately after a glass of water and honey.

Spasms, gastric: When the pains occur, five drops on a little brown sugar. Take immediately after a large glass of water and honey.

Worms (oxyures): See Emmenagogue.

External uses
Insect bites and stings: A little pure essence on the sting.

Verrucae and warts: See Insect bites and stings.

SASSAFRAS
(Sassafras officinale)

Active principles
The essence is obtained from the roots and bark of the sassafras by steam distillation. It contains mainly safril (up to 80 per cent), camphor, eugenol, phellandrene, and pinene.

Properties
Carminative. Diaphoretic. Diuretic. Stimulant. Sudorific.

External uses
Insect bites and stings: Apply a drop of essence to the sting.

Rheumatism: Rub with 90° alcohol and 6 per cent of essence of sassafras or with lukewarm olive oil and 10 per cent of essence.

Internal uses
Dermatitis: Bathe with boiled water and 2 per cent of essence. Smear with the following compound: 1000 ml sweet almond oil + 250g white wax + 750 ml distilled water + 25g essence of sassafras.

Exhaustion, mental and physical: Two drops of essence on a little brown sugar before every meal.

Gout: One drop of essence on a little brown sugar after every meal. In addition, rubbing (see Rheumatism under External uses).

Menstruation problems: Two drops of essence on a little brown sugar after every meal.

Rheumatism: See Gout.

SAVORY

(Satureia montana)
Fr. Sarriette   Ger. Bohnenkraut
Pfefferkraut

Active principles
There is winter savory (*Satureia hortensis*), which is highly valued in cooking, and summer savory (*Satureia montana*). Both are very aromatic and yield by distillation an oil containing carvacrol (up to 40 per cent), cymene (up to 25 per cent), and terpenes.

Properties
Antispasmodic. Antiseptic. Antiputrefactive. Scar-forming. Digestive. Expectorant. Stimulant. Vermifuge.

External uses
Otitis: Put a little warm olive oil with 10 per cent essence of savory into the auditory duct. Rub behind the ear with the pure essence.

Wounds: Clean with boiled water and 2 per cent of essence of savory. Brush over with olive oil and 10 per cent of essence of savory.

Internal uses
Aphthae: Mouthwash of lukewarm boiled water with 2 per cent of essence of savory.

Asthma: Four drops of essence on a little brown sugar after every meal.

Bronchitis: See Asthma.

Digestion, slow: See Asthma.

Digestive spasms and diarrhoea: See Asthma. Rub the abdomen with 80° alcohol and 6 per cent of essence of sassafras or with cream (1000 ml sweet almond oil + 250g white wax + 750g distilled water + 25g essence of savory).

Exhaustion, mental and sexual: Five drops of essence on a little brown sugar half-an-hour before every meal.

Throat: See Asthma. In addition, frequent lukewarm gargling. (Pour half a coffee-spoonful of 80° alcohol and 6 per cent of essence of savory into 100 ml of hot distilled water.)

Worms: See Asthma.

TANGERINE

(Citrus nobilis)

Fr. Mandarine   Ger. Zwergapfelsine

Extracted from the peel, essence of tangerine is a laxative and stomachic. It is added to the essences of lemon and orange in order to vary their taste and accentuate their properties.

TARRAGON

(Artemisia dracunculus)

Fr. Estragon   Ger. Estragon

Active principles
Obtained by distillation from the plant, the essential oil contains phellandrene, ocimene, methylchavicol, herniarin (hydroxycoumarin), estragole (up to 60 per cent), and terpenes.

Properties
Internal antiseptic. Antispasmodic. Carminative. Emmenagogue. Stomachic. Vermifuge.

Internal uses
Anorexia (loss of appetite): Four drops of essence on a little brown sugar half-an-hour before meals.

Antisepsis, intestinal: Five drops of essence on a little brown sugar between meals.

Digestion, slow: Four drops of essence on a little brown sugar after every meal.

Flatulence: See Digestion, slow.

Periods, painful or irregular: See Antisepsis, intestinal.

Rheumatism: See Antisepsis, intestinal.

Spasms, gastric: See Digestion, slow.

Worms (oxyures): Five drops of essence three times a day, preferably between meals. Lukewarm enemas with boiled water (300 ml) into which olive oil with 10 per cent of essence of tarragon has been stirred.

N.B. Infusions of tarragon (40g per litre) possess the same properties as the essence but to a weaker extent. They can be made more potent by adding one drop of essence to each cup. The addition of tarragon leaves to raw green salad gives the latter an agreeable aroma and endows it with the qualities of the essential oil. Furthermore, olive or sunflower-seed oil can be used directly with tarragon (1g of essence to the litre).

THYME (GARDEN)

(Thymus vulgaris)

Fr. Thym   Ger. Gartenthymian

Active principles

The essence drawn from the flower-heads by distillation contains thymol, carvacrol, cymene, pinenes, borneol, linalool.

Properties

Aperitive. Intestinal, pulmonary, and renal antiseptic. Antispasmodic. Balsamic. Carminative. Diuretic. Emmenagogue. Expectorant. Flatulence. Hypertensive. Leucocyte stimulant. Stomachic. Sudorific. Tonic.

External uses

Fatigue: Bathing. Pour into a bath 300g of bicarbonate of soda impregnated with the following oleaginous mixture: 3g essence of thyme + 2g essence of lavender + 1g essence of rosemary.

Rheumatism: Rubbing with 80° alcohol and 6 per cent of essence of thyme. Rubbing with olive oil, 10 per cent of essence of thyme, and 5 per cent of essence of lemon.

Skin: See Fatigue. Wash with boiled water and 2 per cent of essence of thyme. Smear with the following compound: 1000 ml olive oil + 250g white wax + 750 ml distilled water + 10g essence of lemon + 20g essence of thyme.

Vaginitis: Douche of boiled water with 2 per cent of essence of thyme.

Internal uses

Anaemia: Three drops of essence on a little brown sugar half-an-hour before each meal.

Asthma: See Throat, sore.

Chlorosis: See Anaemia.

Coughs: See Throat, sore.

Digestion, slow: See Flatulence. Rub the abdomen with 80° alcohol and 6 per cent of essence.

Emphysema: See Asthma.

Exhaustion, mental and physical: See Anaemia. Rub the spinal column with 80° alcohol and 6 per cent of essence or with olive oil and 10 per cent of essence.

Fevers: See Flatulence.

Flatulence: Three drops of essence on a little brown sugar after each meal.

Hypotension: See Flatulence.

Influenza: See Anaemia.

Leucorrhoea: See Anaemia. Lukewarm douches of boiled water with 2 per cent of essence of thyme.

Periods, scanty: See Leucorrhoea.

Throat, sore: See Anaemia. In addition, gargling with lukewarm boiled water and 2 per cent of essence.

Worms: See Flatulence. Enema (300 ml of boiled water into which has been stirred a soup-spoonful of olive oil with 5 per cent of essence of thyme).

N.B. In aromatherapy, we avoid substituting thymol for essence of thyme. For some people the former can be toxic.

THYME (WILD)
(Thymus serpyllum)
Fr. Serpolet   Ger. Kleiner Kostets

Active principles
The essential oil of wild thyme contains thymol, cymol, and carvacrol. It is very similar to garden thyme.

Properties
Very similar to those of garden thyme. Antispasmodic. Disinfectant. Expectorant. Digestive stimulant. Tonic.

Uses
Much the same as those of garden thyme. These two essences are often partnered in prescriptions in the proportion of two parts of essence of garden thyme to one of essence of wild thyme.

TURMERIC
(Curcuma longa)
Fr. Curry   Ger. Gelbwurzel

Active principles
The rhizome contains an essential oil rich in ketonic turmerone, a resin, and a yellow colouring matter (curcumin) which may, through abuse over a long period, cause a hyperacid stomach and sometimes ulcers.

Properties
Cholagogue. Digestive. Diuretic. Laxative. Liver ailments.

External use
Pains in the bones: Rubbing with lukewarm sweet almond oil and 5 per cent of oil of turmeric.

Internal uses
Anorexia: Half an hour before a meal, two drops of essence on a little brown sugar.

Digestion, slow: After a meal, two drops of essence on a little brown sugar.

Liver, sluggish: See Digestion, slow.

N.B. The essential oil of turmeric must be used in moderation and with care for a fairly limited period. The same applies to rhizome-based tisanes.

TURPENTINE

The essences of turpentine are essential oils extracted from the resins of conifers and *Anacardiaceae* by distillation (predominantly terebenthene).

Active principles
Terpenes, terebenthene.

Properties
Antispasmodic. Antirheumatic. Dissolves biliary calculi. Pulmonary and genito-urinary antiseptic. Haemostatic. Counter-irritant. Parasiticide.

External use
Throat: Inhalations. Pour a coffee-spoonful of the following mixture into 100 ml of boiling water: 1000 ml alcohol + 60g essence of eucalyptus + 60g essence of pine.

Internal uses
Bronchitis: Two capsules of essence, each of 0.25g, twice a day.

Colitis: Three capsules between meals (daily total: six).

Constipation: About ten capsules of essence spread over the day.

Dropsy: See Colitis.

Epilepsy: See Colitis.

Fever, puerperal: Four capsules between meals (daily total: eight).

Flatulence: See Colitis.

Haemoptysis: See Fever, puerperal (if necessary, increase the dose to twelve capsules of essence spread over the full day).

Leucorrhoea: See Colitis.

Migraine: At the most, six capsules of essence spread over the whole day.

Tuberculosis: See Fever, puerperal.

Whooping cough: See Bronchitis. For children between five and ten years, reduce by half.

Worms, intestinal: See Haemoptysis.

VALERIAN
(Valeriana officinalis)
Fr. Valériane   Ger. Baldrian

Active principles
Extracted from the roots of the rhizome, the essential oil contains volatile esters, bornyl-isovalerianate, butyrate, and also alkaloids (chatinine and valerene).

Properties
Sedative. Digestive.

Internal uses
Digestive disorders: Four drops of essence on a little

brown sugar after every meal. Some people prefer two drops of essence of valerian and two drops of essence of lemon.

Hysteria: Three drops of essence on a little brown sugar between meals.

Migraine: See Hysteria.

Nervous disorders: See Digestive disorders.

Neurasthenia: See Hysteria.

VERBENA (LEMON-GRASS)
(Andropogon citratus)
Fr. Verveine Indienne   Ger. Eisenkraut

Active principles
Obtained by distillation, the essence contains citrol in particular.

Properties
Antiseptic. Galactogen. Digestive. Parasiticide.

External use
Pediculosis: Ointment – 1000 ml olive oil + 250g white wax + 750g distilled water + 10g essence of thyme + 20g essence of verbena.

Internal uses
Digestion, difficult: Five drops of essence on a little brown sugar after each meal.

Enteritis: See digestion, difficult.

Milk, insufficient: See Digestion, difficult.

YLANG-YLANG

(Anona odorantissima) and *(Cananga odorata)*

Active principles

Obtained by steam distillation from the flowers of Reunion or Philippines ylang-ylang, the essence contains eugenol, geraniol, linalool, safrol, pinene, terpenes, cadinene, benzoate of benzyl, and more or less esterified acids – acetic, benzoic, formic, salicylic, valerianic – and ylangol (terpenic alcohol), etc.

Properties

Antiseptic. Sedative. Hypotensive. Regulates cardiac and respiratory rhythm.

Internal uses

Frigidity: Five drops of essence on a little brown sugar after every meal.

Hypertension: Three drops of essence on a little brown sugar after every meal.

Infections, intestinal: See Frigidity.

Lung trouble: See Hypertension.

Tachycardia: See Hypertension.

CHAPTER FOUR

AROMATIC WATERS

These are not just dilute alcohol solutions, such as eau-de-Cologne, but are essentially pure distilled water to which is added one or more of the foregoing essences.

Generally speaking, 2g of essential oil is added per litre (20° average solubility). Shake well and often in a glass bottle for two days, then strain and keep in a cool place. In this way we obtain water of anise, basil, borneol, chamomile, caraway, centaury, cinnamon, citron, coriander, cypress, eucalyptus, fennel, garlic, gentian, geranium, goosefoot, hyssop, juniper, laurel, lavender, lemon, marjoram, melissa, niaouli, nutmeg, onion, orange (Seville), origanum, peppermint, rosemary, sage, santolina, sassafras, savory, tangerine, tarragon, turmeric, verbena, ylang-ylang.

On average, a liqueur glass (30 ml) of aromatic water corresponds to three drops of concentrated essence, and on this basis three drops of essence on sugar can be replaced by an aromatic water, which itself can be sweetened. Aromatic water is also a useful alternative to the alcohol preparations, especially where children are involved.

Aromatized water can be kept for a long time in a corked glass bottle, away from the light, and at a temperature of 10°-15°C (50°-60°F). In some cases, distilled water can be replaced by a slightly mineral Evian-type water.

INFUSIONS AND TISANES

In the same way, the infusions and tisanes prescribed by phytotherapists can be enriched, after sweetening them and before drinking them, by a drop of the essence corresponding to the plant. By this means, the potency of the beverage is enhanced while the essential oil is harmonized and somewhat de-artificialized.

Where an exact aromatherapeutic treatment is involved, the cup can take two or three drops of essence. The important thing is to stir the liquid well before drinking it.

AROMATHERAPEUTIC PROPORTIONS

If we take as an average basis two grams of essential oil dissolved in one litre of pure water, that is about one hundred drops of the essence. Hence the following correspondences:

Drops	Water
100 (2 grams)	for 1000 ml
10	for 100 ml
7	for 70 ml (one small glassful)
3	for 30 ml (one liqueur glassful)
1	for 10 ml (one dessertspoonful)

MICROBICIDAL POWER OF CERTAIN ESSENCES

When dissolved in pure water, many of the essential oils have great bactericidal power in doses between 0.2 and 2 per cent. For example, in a concentration of 0.18 per cent essence of cloves kills the tubercular bacillus in a few minutes. This action occurs without damaging the tissues and without poisoning the organism – a risk run by many pharmaceutical preparations and many antibiotics.

Whether introduced into the human body via the skin (alcohol preparations, aromatized oils, cold cream, ointments), via the mouth, or via the nose (inhalations, perfumes) essential oils spread throughout the organic whole before being at least partly expelled by the lungs, sweat, or urine. It is truly a question of a tissue embalmment which is both complete and without danger in the doses used.

ELECTUARIES

Essences are conveyed not only by water (saturation in weak doses), by brown sugar, honey, alcohol, vegetable oils, animal and vegetable fats, cold cream, sodium bicarbonate, but also by electuaries. Among these, that of juniper is highly advantageous. Reduce dried juniper berries to a fine powder. Incorporate them with some pure honey in equal proportions. Allow to cook gently while stirring. Let it cool slowly, continuing to stir, and, to incorporate the essential oil, pour it drop by drop. In the case of essence of lemon or cinnamon, the number of drops corresponds to one per dessertspoonful of electuary. Once the cooling has been completed, the mass keeps well. Take a coffee-spoonful now and again for a daily total of about ten spoonsful. It is very effective in anaemia, for stomach pains, palpitations, dizzy spells, and loss of appetite.

SPICED WINES

In the past when essential oil extractions did not generally exist, and at present for people to whom they are not available, spiced wines were and still are good aromatherapeutic measures. For example, allow 20g of cinnamon, 1g of cloves, 4g of ginger, 5g of nutmeg, and 2g of cardamom to infuse for a week in a litre of good-quality wine with the addition of 300g of brown sugar. Strain. Take a liqueur-glassful (30 ml) a quarter of an hour before each meal. This aperitif stimulates the stomach and heart and purifies the alimentary canal. Don't abuse it.

VINEGARS

Wine or cider vinegars are sometimes used as media for essences, especially for physical care.

Antiseptic vinegar (widely used for skin complaints): 70g white vinegar + 10g solid acetic acid + 3g essence of cloves + 10g essence of lemon + 8g essence of lavender + 3g essence of aspic.

Vinaigre des quatre voleurs (prevention of infectious illnesses): Dissolve 16g of borneol in 125g of crystallized acetic acid. In addition, let the following macerate for a fortnight in four litres of very strong white vinegar: 8g clove of garlic + 8g nutmeg + 8g cloves + 8g cinnamon bark + 48g heads of sage + 48g heads of rue + 48g rosemary + 48g mint + 64g lavender + 96g mugwort. Squeeze and strain. Mix the two liquids. Strain again.

Vinaigre d'Hébé (for freckles): 6600g distilled vinegar + 850g 90° alcohol + 800g distilled water + 60g essence of lemon + 60g essence of citron + 250g essence of lavender. Expose to sunlight for three days. Strain.

Pure white vinegar (a few drops when washing to tone up the skin): 80° alcohol + white vinegar + tincture of benzoin (in equal parts). Leave for three days. Filter. Makes the water for washing milky and perfumes it.

Aromatic vinegar (for inhaling in case of indisposition, fainting, dizziness): 1000g solid acetic acid + 250g Borneo camphor + 4g essence of cinnamon + 3g essence of lavender + 10g essence of cloves. Leave for three days. Strain.

CHAPTER FIVE

DISEASES AND AROMATIC TREATMENTS

For each disease, the names of the plants used in phytotherapy are given in small letters, simply for information and comparison; the names of the essential oils are in capital letters, which are italicized when the plant itself is employed in phytotherapy and its essence in aromatherapy.

Abdominal distension: GARLIC, angelica, *ANISE*, mugwort, CHAMOMILE, CINNAMON, carrot, CARAWAY, CORIANDER, TARRAGON, *FENNEL*, GINGER, CLOVE, HYSSOP, LAVENDER, MARJORAM, melissa, MINT, NUTMEG, ONION, PINE, ROSEMARY, savory.

Abscesses, cold: GARLIC, plantain.

Abscesses, hot: ONION, sweet woodruff, borage.

Aches and pains, muscular: LAVENDER, THYME.

Acid, uric (in excess): LEMON, JUNIPER.

Acne: Burdock, CAJEPUT, JUNIPER, LAVENDER, wild pansy.

Acne rosacea: LAVENDER.

Adenitis: GARLIC, ONION, PINE, ROSEMARY, SAGE.

Adipose tissue: LEMON, ONION, meadowsweet, willow, elder.

Aerophagy: ANISE, *CARAWAY*, LEMON, CORIANDER, TARRAGON, fennel, MARJORAM, *MINT, ORIGANS*, veronica.

Ageing: GARLIC, LEMON, JUNIPER, LAVENDER, ONION, THYME.

Albuminuria: JUNIPER, ONION.

Alopecia (massage): Arnica, burdock, birch, *LAVENDER*, nettle, meadowsweet, rosemary, soapwort, *SAGE*, marigold, tormentil, *THYME*.

Amenorrhoea: Milfoil, mugwort, elecampane, *CHAMOMILE, MINT,* buckbean, *ORIGANS,* parsley, *SAGE*, marigold, THYME, CLOVE.

Anaemia: GARLIC, MUGWORT, elecampane, CHAMOMILE, carrot, knapweed, cabbage, LEMON, scurvy-grass, cress, strawberry, *GENTIAN,* buckbean, nettle, parsley, horseradish, *THYME.*

Anal fistulas: LEMON, LAVENDER, NIAOULI.

Anasarca: See Dropsy.

Angina pectoris: Hawthorn, *ANISE.*

Anorexia: See Appetite, loss of.

Anosmia: See Smell, loss of sense of.

Antiseptics: GARLIC, BORNEOL, CINNAMON, EUCALYPTUS, JUNIPER, CLOVE, LAVENDER, NIAOULI, PINE, ROSEMARY, THYME, YLANG-YLANG.

Anxiety: Hawthorn, LAVENDER, MARJORAM, melissa, savory, *VALERIAN.*

Anxiety attacks: Hawthorn, BASIL, dog-rose.

Aphonia: CYPRESS.

Aphthae: Self-heal, *CHAMOMILE, LEMON,* oak, mountain avens, *GERANIUM,* bilberry, walnut, nettle, potentilla, *ROSEMARY*, blackberry, *SAGE, THYME,* violet.

Apoplexy: Mustard, horse-radish, LAVENDER.

Appetite, loss of: Angelica, ANISE, BERGAMOT, CHAMOMILE, carline, *CARAWAY,* common centaury, knapweed, chicory, LEMON, CORIANDER, TARRAGON, fennel, JUNIPER, ginger, HYSSOP, horehound, melissa, NUTMEG, *ORIGANS,* dandelion, SAGE.

Arteriosclerosis: GARLIC, hawthorn, LEMON, greater celandine, JUNIPER, ONION, wild pansy, horse-tail, rue, sunflower.

Arthritis: GARLIC, globe artichoke, white bryony, rest-harrow, century, knapweed, couch grass, ash, *JUNIPER*, ONION, horsetail, meadowsweet, golden rod, starwort, elder.

Ascites: LEMON, cabbage, *ONION*, meadowsweet.

Asthma: Wild celery, GARLIC, ANISE, mullein, bryony, CAJEPUT, LEMON, red poppy, sundew, EUCALYPTUS, HYSSOP, *LAVENDER*, ground ivy, lobelia, horehound, *MELISSA*, MINT, St John's wort, ONION, ORIGANS, *ROSEMARY, SAVORY, SAGE,* wild thyme, *GARDEN THYME,* coltsfoot, valerian, garlic-mustard.

Atony, gastric: Agrimony, GARLIC, *MUGWORT,* herb bennet, carline, *CARAWAY,* common centaury, chicory, fennel, gentian, melissa, *MINT,* SAGE, *THYME,* dill.

Azotaemia (excess of urea in the blood): JUNIPER, ONION.

Backache: CHAMOMILE, GERANIUM, LAVENDER.

Bed-wetting: See Enuresis.

Bilious attack: LAVENDER, MINT, VERBENA.

Bleeding: See Haemorrhage.

Blepharitis: Sweet woodruff, *CHAMOMILE,* LEMON, greater celandine, parsley.

Blisters: Marsh mallow, LAVENDER.

Blood-pressure, high: See Hypertension.

Blood-pressure, low: See Hypotension.

Boils: See Furunculosis.

Breast-feeding: ANISE, CARAWAY, *FENNEL,* goat's rue, nettle, *VERBENA.* To dry up the milk: *SAGE.*

Breasts (see Chapping): CHAMOMILE, comfrey, tansy.

Breasts, congestion of: Milfoil, chervil, fennel, GERANIUM, *MINT,* parsley.

Breath, bad: MINT.

Bronchitis, acute: Wild celery, GARLIC, angelica, elecampane, burdock, mullein, borage, CAJEPUT, LEMON, EUCALYPTUS, HYSSOP, LAVENDER, MINT, ONION, PINE, THYME, garlic-mustard.

Bronchitis, chronic: Wild celery, GARLIC, angelica, mullein, borage, CAJEPUT, maidenhair fern, lady's smock, carrot, chervil, LEMON, comfrey, red poppy, cress, sundew, EUCALYPTUS, marsh mallow, HYSSOP, LAVENDER, ground ivy, horehound, mallow, melissa, MINT, NIAOULI, ONION, ORIGANS, PINE, oak fern, primula, horseradish, liquorice, ROSEMARY, SANDAL-WOOD, savory, SAGE, thyme, coltsfoot, violet.

Brucellosis: See Fever, Malta.

Bruises: See Contusions.

Burns and scalds: CHAMOMILE, carrot, comfrey, EUCALYPTUS, GERANIUM, LAVENDER, St John's wort, NIAOULI, onion, ROSEMARY, SAGE, marigold.

Buzzing in the ears: Hawthorn, ONION, black horehound.

Capillaries, fragile: LEMON.

Cellulitis: ORIGANS, meadowsweet.

Change of Life: See Menopause.

Chapping and frost-bite: CHAMOMILE, LEMON, ONION, tansy, garlic-mustard.

Chilblains: Knapweed, LEMON, LAVENDER, ONION, marigold.

Childbirth (to prepare for and facilitate): Comfrey, goat's rue, CLOVE, laurel, horehound, wild pansy, violet.

Children's illnesses: LEMON

Chills: EUCALYPTUS, LAVENDER, PINE, THYME.

Chlorosis: LAVENDER, PINE, ROSEMARY, THYME.

Cholecystitis: Greater celandine. See Lithiasis, biliary.

Cholera: CINNAMON, EUCALYPTUS, MINT.

Cholesterol: Globe artichoke, JUNIPER, ROSEMARY.

Cirrhosis: Cabbage, JUNIPER, ONION, ROSEMARY.

Colds: LAVENDER, MARJORAM, NIAOULI, borage, *ONION*, oak fern, liquorice, *THYME*, coltsfoot, violet. See Bronchitis.

Colds, chronic: GARLIC, BASIL, LAVENDER.

Colibacillosis: Sweet woodruff, heather, CORIANDER, EUCALYPTUS, SANDALWOOD.

Colic, hepatic: Flax. See Lithiasis, biliary.

Colic, intestinal: GARLIC, ANISE, BERGAMOT, mullein, caraway, red poppy, HYSSOP, MINT, onion.

Colic, renal: Couch-grass, flax, mallow. See Lithiasis, urinary.

Colitis: ROSEMARY, VERBENA.

Conjunctivitis: Sweet woodruff, *CHAMOMILE*, LEMON, greater celandine, parsley.

Constipation: Bryony, chamomile, dog-rose, flax, mallow, oak fern, ROSEMARY, white roses, wild thyme, violet.

Contagious diseases (protection): *GARLIC*, EUCALYPTUS, JUNIPER, CLOVE.

Contusions: Arnica, bryony, CINNAMON, hyssop, *LAVENDER*, flax, mint, St John's wort, primula, *ROSEMARY*, SAGE, marigold, thyme.

Convalescence: BORNEOL, cardamom, carrot, centaury, cabbage, LEMON, dog-rose, buckbean, NUTMEG, parsley, *ROSEMARY, SAGE, THYME*.

Convulsions: Mugwort, CHAMOMILE, valerian.

Corns: GARLIC, greater celandine, *ONION*.

Coryza: See Colds.

Coughs: GARLIC, ANISE, elecampane, red poppy, HYSSOP, LAVENDER, mallow, MINT, ONION, ORIGANS, liquorice, WILD THYME, GARDEN THYME, coltsfoot.

Coughs, convulsive: CYPRESS, EUCALYPTUS, LAVENDER, ORIGANS, PINE, THYME.

Cracked skin: ONION.
Cystitis: Mullein, heather, CAJEPUT, EUCALYPTUS, JUNIPER, LAVENDER, flax, mallow, St John's wort, NIAOULI, PINE, SANDALWOOD, doradilla.

Deafness: GARLIC, fennel, NIAOULI, ONION, SAVORY.
Debility: GARLIC, BORNEOL, CINNAMON, LEMON, EUCALYPTUS, JUNIPER, GERANIUM, GINGER, CLOVE, HYSSOP, LAVENDER, MINT, NUTMEG, ONION, PINE, ROSEMARY, SAVORY, SAGE, THYME. This wide choice of essential oils enables the treatment to be varied and better adapted to the patient's temperament.
Debility, general (see Debility): Carrot, knapweed, *HYSSOP, LAVENDER, MINT,* buckbean, horseradish, *ROSEMARY, SAGE, THYME.*
Debility, nervous: BASIL.
Depression, nervous: BORNEOL, CHAMOMILE.
Diabetes: Globe artichoke, burdock, EUCALYPTUS, strawberry, JUNIPER, GERANIUM, *ONION.*
Diarrhoea: Agrimony, GARLIC, herb bennet, mullein, *CHAMOMILE,* CINNAMON, carrot, blackcurrant, LEMON, coriander, strawberry plant, JUNIPER, gentian, GERANIUM, ginger, CLOVE, LAVENDER, *MINT,* NUTMEG, *ORANGE,* nettle, burnet, plantain, potentilla, knot-grass, ROSEMARY, blackberry, red rose, SANDALWOOD, savory, *SAGE.*
Disinfection of rooms: EUCALYPTUS, JUNIPER, GERANIUM, LAVENDER, PINE, THYME.
Distension, abdominal: See Abdominal distension.
Diuretics: CYPRESS, JUNIPER, ONION, ROSEMARY, SAGE.
Dizzy spells: ANISE, hawthorn, *CHAMOMILE,* CARAWAY, FENNEL, *LAVENDER,* melissa, *MINT, ROSEMARY, SAGE, THYME.*
Dropsy: GARLIC, sweet woodruff, bryony, greater celandine, cress, *ONION,* parsley, horsetail,

horseradish, meadowsweet, hawkweed, forget-me-not.

Dysentery: GARLIC, BASIL, mullein, CAJEPUT, blackcurrant, LEMON, strawberry plant, horehound, mallow, bilberry, NIAOULI, burnet, knot-grass, THYME.

Dysidrosis: PINE.

Dysmenorrhoea: Shepherd's purse, parsley, SAGE, marigold, ANISE, CHAMOMILE, CARAWAY, LEMON, CYPRESS, TARRAGON, JUNIPER, CLOVE, LAVENDER, MINT, ROSEMARY.

Dyspepsia: Milfoil, GARLIC, ANISE, angelica, mugwort, sweet woodruff, CHAMOMILE, CINNAMON, carrot, centaury, LEMON, CORIANDER, tarragon, fennel, JUNIPER, gentian, CLOVE, HYSSOP, LAVENDER, melissa, mint, ONION, ORIGANS, dandelion, ROSEMARY, SAVORY, SAGE, wild thyme, GARDEN THYME, VERBENA, dill.

Dyspepsia, atonic: JUNIPER, GINGER, LAVENDER, NUTMEG, ORIGANS, ROSEMARY, SAGE, THYME.

Dyspepsia, nervous: CARAWAY, ORANGE, SEVILLE ORANGE.

Dyspnoea: HYSSOP

Dystonia, neurovegetative: TARRAGON, LAVENDER, ORIGANS, ROSEMARY, VERBENA.

Earache: GARLIC, CAJEPUT, LAVENDER.

Ecchymoses (see Contusions): Fennel, *HYSSOP*, primula.

Eczema: Burdock, CHAMOMILE, carrot, greater celandine, HYSSOP, wild pansy, SAGE.

Eczema, dry: JUNIPER, LAVENDER.

Eczema, weeping: JUNIPER.

Emmenagogues: ROSEMARY, SAGE, THYME.

Emphysema: GARLIC, EUCALYPTUS, THYME.

Enteritis: CAJEPUT, CHAMOMILE, GERANIUM,

LAVENDER, bilberry, NIAOULI, nettle, burnet, knot-grass, VERBENA.

Enuresis: CYPRESS, PINE.

Epidemics (prevention of): GARLIC, LEMON, EUCALYPTUS, JUNIPER, LAVENDER, NIAOULI, PINE, THYME.

Epistaxis: LEMON, LAVENDER, PINE.

Erethism, cardiovascular: ANISE, CARAWAY.

Erysipelas: Chervil, *WILD THYME.*

Exophthalmic goitre: See Goitre, exophthalmic.

Eyelids (inflammation): CHAMOMILE, LEMON, plantain, tea.

Fainting fits: CINNAMON, melissa, MINT, ROSEMARY.

Feet, sensitive: LEMON, EUCALYPTUS, PINE.

Ferments, intestinal: Dill, TARRAGON, JUNIPER, CLOVE, *MINT, ONION, ORIGANS*, savory, *WILD THYME, GARDEN THYME.*

Feverish conditions: LEMON, EUCALYPTUS, LAVENDER, THYME.

Fever, Malta: EUCALYPTUS, LAVENDER, PINE, THYME.

Fever, rheumatic: ORIGANS, PINE.

Fevers, intermittent and nervous: Wild celery, garlic, borage, CHAMOMILE, knapweed, *LAVENDER*, horehound, *ROSEMARY, SAGE*, violet.

Fevers with rash: EUCALYPTUS, HYSSOP, LAVENDER.

Fistulas, anal: See Anal fistulas.

Flatulence (see Abdominal distension): Dill, angelica, ANISE, mugwort, carrot, fennel, melissa, savory, *THYME.*

Flu: See Influenza.

Fractures (to help the bone to knit): Horsetail.

Freckles: LEMON, MINT, ONION, parsley.

Frigidity: See Impotence.

Furunculosis: Arnica, burdock, hogweed, mullein,

CHAMOMILE, LEMON, marsh mallow, *ONION*, plantain, potentilla, tormentil, marigold, *THYME*.

Gastritis: LEMON.
General debility: See Debility, general.
Gingivitis: See Gums.
Glossitis: LEMON, GERANIUM, liquorice, SAGE.
Goitre, exophthalmic: GARLIC, ONION.
Gout: External treatments – Burdock, bryony, *CHAMOMILE, LAVENDER*, St John's wort, *ROSEMARY, SAGE.* Internal treatments – GARLIC, burdock, BASIL, CAJEPUT, *CHAMOMILE*, cabbage, LEMON, fennel, JUNIPER, *LAVENDER*, St John's wort, PINE, *ROSEMARY*.
Growth: LEMON, JUNIPER, ONION.
Gums (weakness of): Herb bennet, LEMON, CLOVE, LAVENDER, SAGE, THYME.

Haematuria: LEMON, strawberry plant, burnet, horsetail, knot-grass, milk-thistle.
Haemoptysis: Milfoil, CINNAMON, comfrey, CYPRESS, JUNIPER, GERANIUM, laurel, nettle, PINE, plantain, horsetail.
Haemorrhage, gastric: Shepherd's purse, LEMON, nettle, horsetail, blackberry, red roses, *WILD THYME*, milk-thistle.
Haemorrhage, intestinal: LEMON, nettle, burnet, PINE, plantain, potentilla, horsetail, knot-grass, blackberry, red roses, *WILD THYME*, milk-thistle.
Haemorrhage, nasal: See Epistaxis.
Haemorrhage, pulmonary: See Haemoptysis.
Haemorrhage, uterine: CINNAMON, CYPRESS, JUNIPER, GERANIUM, PINE.
Haemorrhoids: Milfoil, GARLIC, mullein, goosefoot, couchgrass, CYPRESS, ONION, horsetail, snakeweed, milk-thistle.
Hair: See Alopecia. Care – Nettle, SAGE, THYME.
Halitosis: See Breath, bad.

Hands (keeping smooth): LEMON.

Headache: LEMON, lavender, feverfew, chamomile, melissa, MINT, buckbean.

Head cold: See Colds.

Head noises: See Buzzing in the ears.

Hearing, loss of: See Deafness.

Heart (nervous heart trouble): Hawthorn, olive, ROSEMARY.

Heartburn (acidity): *LEMON,* comfrey, hops, flax, melilot, melissa, *MINT,* bog myrtle, valerian, masterwort.

Herpes (see also Skin diseases): Elecampane, burdock, CHAMOMILE, carline, carrot, greater celandine, LEMON, GERANIUM, nightshade, dandelion.

Herpes (of the mucous membranes): LEMON.

Hiccups: Dill, *ANISE,* TARRAGON, valerian.

Hives: See Urticaria.

Hoarseness: Garlic-mustard, cabbage, CYPRESS, horseradish.

Hookworms: GOOSEFOOT, THYME.

Hypertension: GARLIC, hawthorn, hogweed, greater celandine, LEMON, strawberry, olive, SAGE, YLANG-YLANG.

Hyperviscosity of the blood: LEMON.

Hypotension: Hawthorn, LEMON, olive, milk-thistle.

Hysteria: CAJEPUT, LAVENDER, ROSEMARY, valerian.

Icterus: Agrimony, globe artichoke, chervil, greater celandine, LEMON, GERANIUM, dandelion, ROSEMARY.

Impetigo (see Skin diseases): Garlic-mustard, burdock, wild pansy, marigold.

Impotence: Hogweed, CINNAMON, CLOVE, *MINT,* ONION, PINE, ROSEMARY, SANDALWOOD, *SAVORY,* YLANG-YLANG.

Incontinence of urine: See Enuresis.

Indigestion: CARAWAY, LAVENDER, melissa, *MINT.*

Infection, intestinal: BASIL, bilberry, ROSEMARY, SAGE, THYME, YLANG-YLANG.

Infection, puerperal: LAVENDER, NIAOULI.

Infections: GARLIC, BORNEOL, LEMON, CLOVE, LAVENDER, MINT.

Infection, urinary (see Cystitis): EUCALYPTUS, JUNIPER, NIAOULI, ONION, PINE THYME.

Infectious diseases: GARLIC, BORNEOL, EUCALYPTUS, CLOVE, LAVENDER, THYME.

Inflammations: Mullein, borage, *CHAMOMILE,* marsh mallow, mallow, liquorice.

Influenza: GARLIC, elecampane, borage, *CHAMOMILE,* CINNAMON, LEMON, CYPRESS, dog-rose, EUCALYPTUS, fennel, HYSSOP, *LAVENDER,* MINT, NIAOULI, *ONION, PINE,* primula, *ROSEMARY,* SAGE, marigold, *THYME.*

Insect bites and stings: GARLIC, burdock, BASIL, CINNAMON, LEMON, LAVENDER, mallow, *ONION,* parsley, plantain, SAGE, THYME.

Insomnia: Sweet woodruff, hawthorn, black horehound, BASIL, CHAMOMILE, red poppy, dog-rose, MARJORAM, melissa, *MINT,* ORANGE, BERGAMOT, THYME, valerian.

Instability, mental: LAVENDER, MARJORAM.

Intestines (colitis, infections, irritations): GARLIC, CORIANDER, HYSSOP, JUNIPER, LAVENDER, MINT, NIAOULI, THYME, VERBENA, YLANG-YLANG.

Irritability: ANISE, hawthorn, *CHAMOMILE,* CARAWAY, CYPRESS, cheese-rennet, LAVENDER, melissa, *MINT,* olive, *SAGE,* valerian.

Itching: See Scabies.

Jaundice (see Icterus): Agrimony, globe artichoke, greater celandine, chicory, oak fern, dandelion.

Laryngitis (see Throat): *LAVENDER,* NIAOULI, ONION.

Laryngitis, chronic: CAJEPUT, EUCALYPTUS, *LAVENDER,* NIAOULI, ONION, liquorice.

Lassitude, general: See Debility.

Leucorrhoea (see Whites): Mugwort, elecampane, JUNIPER, HYSSOP, laurel, *LAVENDER,* horehound, nettle, *PINE,* potentilla, snakeweed, *ROSEMARY,* blackberry, red rose, *SAGE, THYME.*

Lithiasis, biliary (see Liver ailments in general): Agrimony, globe artichoke, chicory, LEMON, NUTMEG, ONION, PINE, dandelion, ROSEMARY.

Lithiasis, urinary: Wild celery, GARLIC, burdock, heather, blackcurrant, greater celandine, chicory, LEMON, hawkweed, forget-me-not, fennel, JUNIPER, GERANIUM, HYSSOP, mallow, horsetail, horseradish, doradilla.

Liver (see Liver ailments in general): Agrimony, globe artichoke, elecampane, chervil, greater celandine, chicory, *MINT,* buckbean, dandelion, *ROSEMARY.*

Liver ailments (in general): Wild celery, agrimony, globe artichoke, elecampane, chervil, greater celandine, LEMON, cress, *MINT,* buckbean, oak fern, dandelion, *ROSEMARY.*

Liver, congestion of: Globe artichoke, CHAMOMILE, LEMON, buckbean, *ROSEMARY.*

Lungs: See Pleurisy, Pneumonia, Lung troubles.

Lung troubles: GARLIC, CAJEPUT, CYPRESS, *EUCALYPTUS,* fennel, *CLOVE,* HYSSOP, *LAVENDER, MINT,* NIAOULI, *ONION, PINE,* SAGE, *TURPENTINE, THYME.*

Lymphatism: ANISE, CARAWAY, CLOVE, LAVENDER, ONION, ROSEMARY, SAGE.

Malaria: GARLIC, BORNEOL, LEMON, EUCALYPTUS.

Malta fever: See Fever, Malta.

Measles: EUCALYPTUS, LAVENDER, THYME.

Melancholia: LAVENDER.

Memory (loss of): CLOVE, ROSEMARY.

Meningitis: ONION.

Menopause: Hawthorn, black horehound, CHAMOMILE, CYPRESS, SAGE.

Menstruation, difficult: CARAWAY, FENNEL, EUCALYPTUS, JUNIPER, CLOVE, SANTOLINA, SASSAFRAS, SAGE.

Mental instability: See Instability, mental.

Metritis: Comfrey, JUNIPER, HYSSOP, LAVENDER, ROSEMARY, SAGE, THYME.

Metrorrhagia (uterine bleeding): Shepherd's purse, CINNAMON, CYPRESS, JUNIPER, GERANIUM, dead nettle, stinging nettle, PINE, horsetail, milk-thistle.

Migraine: Pasque-flower, angelica, ANISE, *BASIL,* CHAMOMILE, LEMON, EUCALYPTUS, cheese-rennet, *LAVENDER,* MARJORAM, melissa, *MINT,* NUTMEG, ONION, PINE, primula, ROSEMARY, valerian.

Migraine, digestive: ANISE.

Milk (see Breast-feeding): Dill, *ANISE,* fennel.

Milk (cessation of breast-feeding): Chervil, MINT, SAGE.

Minerals in body, decrease of: LEMON.

Mosquitoes (for repelling them): CEDAR, EUCALYPTUS, MINT, ONION, tomato plant. Paint exposed areas with: 80 per cent alcohol and 10 per cent of borneol 40g + 20g essence of cedar + 25g essence of eucalyptus + 10g essence of lemon + 30g essence of verbena.

Muscular aches and pains: See Aches and pains, muscular.

Nails, broken: LEMON.

Nephritis: Wild celery, hawkweed, forget-me-not, fennel, EUCALYPTUS, JUNIPER, GERANIUM, NIAOULI, sea holly, PINE, horsetail, THYME.

Nerves (attack of): Anise, hawthorn, CHAMOMILE, CARAWAY, LAVENDER, melissa, *MINT, SAGE,* THYME, valerian, VERBENA.

Nervous debility: See Debility, nervous.
Nervous depression: See Depression, nervous.
Nervous predisposition: See Nerves.
Nettle-rash: See Urticaria.
Neuralgia: Pasque flower, CHAMOMILE, EUCALYPTUS, *MINT*, PINE, meadowsweet, valerian.
Neuralgia, dental (see Teeth): GARLIC, CAJEPUT, JUNIPER, CLOVE, ONION, SAGE.
Neuralgia, facial: CHAMOMILE, GERANIUM, MINT.
Neuralgia, rheumatoid: CAJEPUT, CHAMOMILE, TARRAGON, EUCALYPTUS, JUNIPER, LAVENDER, MARJORAM, NUTMEG, PINE.
Neurasthenia: LAVENDER, MARJORAM, *SAGE, VERBENA*, valerian.
Nosebleed: See Epistaxis.

Obesity: LEMON, ONION.
Oedema: Bryony, LEMON, ONION, sea holly, horsetail, meadowsweet.
Oliguria: Elecampane, blackcurrant, fennel, JUNIPER, LAVENDER, ONION, SAGE.
Ophthalmia: CHAMOMILE, chervil, greater celandine, GERANIUM, mallow, parsley, plantain, liquorice, marigold, violet.
Otitis: BORNEOL, NIAOULI.
Ovaries (ovarian complaints): CYPRESS.
Over-exertion: Hawthorn, BASIL, centaury, LAVENDER, ONION, *ROSEMARY, SAVORY, SAGE, THYME.*
Oxyures (worms): *GARLIC*, mugwort, CHAMOMILE, GOOSEFOOT, cabbage, EUCALYPTUS, *MINT, ONION*, SANTOLINA, wild thyme, GARDEN THYME, Tansy, scented mayweed.

Palpitations: ANISE, hawthorn, CHAMOMILE, GOOSEFOOT, dog-rose, EUCALYPTUS, melissa, *MINT*, olive, ROSEMARY, santolina, THYME, valerian.

Paralyses: BASIL, JUNIPER, LAVENDER, MINT, ROSEMARY, SAGE.

Pediculosis: CINNAMON, LEMON, EUCALYPTUS, GERANIUM, CLOVE, LAVENDER, ORIGANS, PINE, ROSEMARY, THYME.

Pericarditis: ONION.

Periods: See Dysmenorrhoea.

Periods, painful: See Dysmenorrhoea.

Periods, scanty: Mugwort, BASIL, fennel, LAVENDER, MINT, buckbean, parsley, SANTOLINA, SAGE, marigold.

Phlebitis: ONION.

Piles: See Haemorrhoids.

Plethora: LEMON.

Pleurisy: Angelica, knapweed, horehound, *ONION.*

Pneumonia: Angelica, borage, LEMON, EUCALYPTUS, LAVENDER, horehound, NIAOULI, PINE, primula, marigold.

Pregnancy: Carrot, JUNIPER, LAVENDER, *MELISSA,* SAGE.

Prostate and *Prostatitis:* ONION. (Into a coffee-spoonful of gourd oil pour three drops of essence of onion. To be taken on waking.) PINE.

Pruritus: Elecampane, burdock, *CHAMOMILE, MINT,* THYME.

Puberty: GARLIC, CLOVE, MINT, ONION, PINE, THYME.

Pulse, irregular: See Sinus arrhythmia.

Pulse, rapid: See Tachycardia.

Rheumatic fever: See Fever, rheumatic.

Rheumatism, chronic: GARLIC, burdock, CAJEPUT, *CHAMOMILE,* LEMON, CYPRESS, TARRAGON, EUCALYPTUS, JUNIPER, HYSSOP, *LAVENDER,* St John's wort, *ONION, ORIGANS,* PINE, ROSEMARY, Sassafras, sage, tansy, *THYME.*

Rheumatism, muscular: ORIGANS, PINE, ROSEMARY.

Rhinitis: EUCALYPTUS, LAVENDER, NIAOULI, THYME.

Rickets: Carrot, ONION, parsley, PINE, horsetail, horseradish, *ROSEMARY, THYME.*

Scabies: GARLIC, elecampane, CINNAMON, CARAWAY, LEMON, cheese-rennet, *CLOVE, LAVENDER, MINT,* mustard, ROSEMARY, WILD THYME, GARDEN THYME.

Scalds: See Burns and scalds.

Scarlet fever: See Measles.

Sciatica: Cabbage, St John's wort, PINE, horseradish.

Scrofula: Angelica, centaury, cress, LAVENDER, ONION, parsley.

Scurvy: Lady's smock, LEMON, cabbage, cress, buckbean, *ONION,* parsley.

Secretions, purulent: LEMON, CLOVE, YLANG-YLANG.

Sedatives: ASPIC, CINNAMON, LAVENDER, SAGE.

Shingles: See Zona.

Sinus arrhythmia: Hawthorn, horehound.

Sinusitis: CINNAMON, LEMON, EUCALYPTUS, LAVENDER, NIAOULI, PINE, ROSEMARY, THYME.

Skin (see Skin diseases): LEMON.

Skin, cracked: See Cracked skin.

Skin diseases: Elecampane, burdock, CAJEPUT, CHAMOMILE, carline, chervil, cheese-rennet, marsh mallow, HYSSOP, LAVENDER, nettle, wild pansy, plantain, SASSAFRAS, *THYME.*

Skin eruptions: LEMON, JUNIPER, LAVENDER.

Sleeplessness: See Insomnia.

Smell, loss of sense of: BASIL.

Snake bites, first aid for: BASIL, CINNAMON, LEMON, JUNIPER, CLOVE, LAVENDER, THYME.

Sores, running: Arnica, *LAVENDER,* St John's wort, plantain, knot-grass, *ROSEMARY,* marigold, *THYME.*

Sore throat: Agrimony, blackcurrant, LEMON, strawberry plant, GERANIUM, *HYSSOP*, bilberry, nettle, plantain, potentilla, blackberry, red rose, SAGE, THYME, violet.

Spasms, bronchial: ANISE, CYPRESS, LAVENDER, MARJORAM, PINE.

Spasms, digestive: ANISE, CINNAMON, CORIANDER, LAVENDER, MARJORAM.

Spasms, gastric: GARLIC, angelica, *ANISE*, hawthorn, *BASIL, CAJEPUT, CHAMOMILE, CARAWAY*, greater celandine, *LAVENDER, MARJORAM*, melissa, MINT, buckbean.

Spasms, genital: Pasque flower, EUCALYPTUS, MINT.

Spasms, intestinal: GARLIC, CHAMOMILE, MINT, PINE, liquorice, *SAVORY*.

Spleen, congestion of: CHAMOMILE, borage, *JUNIPER, LAVENDER*.

Sprains (wrenches): Arnica, *LAVENDER, ROSEMARY, SAGE*, tansy, THYME.

Sterility: CINNAMON, JUNIPER, GERANIUM, CLOVE, MINT, SAGE.

Stomach (weak): CARAWAY, CLOVE, ORIGANS, *SAGE, VERBENA*.

Stomach pains: Milfoil, *GARLIC*, CINAMMON, centaury, TARRAGON, fennel, yellow bedstraw, GERANIUM, HYSSOP, horehound, MINT, PINE, ROSEMARY, SAVORY, valerian.

Stomatitis: LEMON, GERANIUM, bilberry, blackberry, *SAGE*.

Sudorifics: Borage, CYPRESS, JUNIPER, hops, *MINT*, elder, *LIME*.

Sweating (of the armpits and hands): Angelica, centaury, horsetail, *SAGE*.

Sweating, profuse: Red rose, *SAGE*.

Tachycardia: Hawthorn, olive, YLANG-YLANG.
Taenia: PINE, THYME.
Tapeworm: See Taenia.

Teeth: CHAMOMILE, teasel, LEMON, CLOVE, origan, parsley, liquorice, *THYME.*

Threadworm: See Worms (ascarides).

Throat (see Sore throat and Tonsillitis): Agrimony, hawthorn, herb bennet, chervil, dog-rose bedeguar, *ORIGAN,* horsetail, *ROSEMARY,* red rose, *SAVORY.*

Throat, sore: See Sore throat.

Thrush: See Aphthae.

Tics: MARJORAM.

Tinea: GARLIC, burdock, LEMON, *LAVENDER.*

Tinnitus: See Buzzing in the ears.

Tonsillitis: Agrimony, hawthorn, chervil, *ORIGAN,* horsetail, *ROSEMARY,* pink rose, *SAVORY.*

Tracheitis: Elecampane, PINE, liquorice, coltsfoot.

Trembling: LAVENDER, MINT, SAGE.

Typhus: EUCALYPTUS, PINE, THYME.

Ulcers (legs): *GARLIC,* JUNIPER, CLOVE, *LAVENDER,* NIAOULI, walnut, ONION, plantain, horsetail, ROSEMARY, SAVORY, SAGE.

Ulcers (stomach, bowel): *GARLIC,* burdock, *CHAMOMILE,* centaury, LEMON, knapweed, greater celandine, cabbage, comfrey, GERANIUM, *LAVENDER,* flax, MINT, *ONION,* nettle, horsetail, ROSEMARY, red rose.

Uraemia: Hawkweed, forget-me-not, hip, JUNIPER, bilberry, ONION, olive, winter cherry.

Uric acid: See Acid, uric.

Urinary tracts: Cress, *EUCALYPTUS,* fennel, *JUNIPER,* GERANIUM, bilberry, NIAOULI, PINE, SANDALWOOD, THYME.

Urticaria: GARLIC, centaury, cabbage, ONION, SAGE, THYME.

Varicose veins: GARLIC, garlic-mustard, shepherd's purse, *LEMON,* cress, *CYPRESS, JUNIPER,* LAVENDER, ONION, olive, parsley, ROSEMARY, marigold.

Verrucae: GARLIC, greater celandine, LEMON, ONION, dandelion, sage.

Vertigo: See Dizzy spells.

Voice: CYPRESS, marsh mallow, flax, mallow, plantain, liquorice, blackberry, THYME, coltsfoot.

Voice, loss of: See Aphonia.

Vomiting: LEMON, MINT, ROSEMARY, SAGE.

Vomiting, nervous: ANISE, CAJEPUT, fennel, MINT.

Warts: See Verrucae.

Whites (see Leucorrhoea): Mugwort, JUNIPER, HYSSOP, dead nettle, *LAVENDER*, horehound, stinging nettle, potentilla, snakeweed, PINE, red rose, *SAGE*, wild thyme, GARDEN THYME.

Whitlow: Mullein, *CHAMOMILE, ONION*, potentilla, tormentil.

Wind: See Flatulence.

Worms (ascarides): *GARLIC, CHAMOMILE,* scented mayweed, *ONION, SANTOLINA*, tansy, OAK FERN, EUCALYPTUS, *MINT*, wild thyme, *GARDEN THYME*.

Worms (oxyures): Mugwort, *GARLIC*, CINNAMON, cabbage, scented mayweed, *MINT, ONION*, PINE, *SANTOLINA*, savory, *WILD THYME*, tansy, *GARDEN THYME*. See also Oxyures.

Wounds: Agrimony, *GARLIC*, garlic-mustard, arnica, CAJEPUT, knapweed, LEMON, COMFREY, dog-rose bedeguar, JUNIPER, GERANIUM, CLOVE, marsh mallow, *LAVENDER, ONION*, plantain, horsetail, red rose, *SAGE*, marigold, *THYME*.

Wounds, atonic: GARLIC, CAJEPUT, comfrey, JUNIPER, CLOVE, *LAVENDER*, NIAOULI, *ONION*, plantain, potentilla, horsetail, ROSEMARY, *SAVORY, SAGE*.

Wounds, infected: GARLIC, LEMON, EUCALYPTUS, JUNIPER, CLOVE, *LAVENDER*, ONION, PINE, *ROSEMARY*, THYME.

Wounds, suppurating: See Wounds, infected.

Wrinkles, facial: LEMON.

Zona: Centaury, cabbage, *LEMON*, horsetail, sarsaparilla, golden rod.

N.B. The above-mentioned essences for each disease are not restrictive. They figure only as examples. Valid also are others which are cited in this book's list of plants with their commonest applications. The reader is requested to consult them.

GLOSSARY

A

adenitis: inflammation of lymph nodes.

aerophagy: swallowing of air.

aldehyde: a compound differing from an alcohol in having two atoms less of hydrogen.

allicine: a water-soluble oil, the principal antibacterial constituent of oil of onion.

allyl: an organic radical, the sulphide of which occurs in oil of garlic. A highly volatile liquid with a pungent odour.

alphapinene: the chief constituent of oil of turpentine, eucalyptus, juniper, etc.

Anacardiaceae: the cashew family of trees and shrubs with gummy, milky, or resinous saps.

anasarca: a generalised form of dropsy.

anethole: the chief constituent of oil of aniseed.

angelicin: a constituent of the roots of *Angelica officinalis*.

Anonaceae: the pineapple family.

anthranilic ester: a compound formed by the union of alcohols and anthranilic acid with elimination of water.

anticarious: arresting dental decay.

antifermentescible: preventing from being capable of fermentation.

antiphlogistic: (medicine) that counteracts inflammation.

antisclerous: preventing sclerosis.

antiureal: preventing the formation of excessive urea.

aphthae: thrush, a disease marked by whitish blisters in mouth and throat.

arbutin: a glucoside (q.v.) obtained from the bearberry and used as a diuretic (q.v.).

aromatherapy: the use of aromatic plants and their essential oils for healing purposes.

ascarides: roundworms.

ascaridol: the active constituent of oil of goosefoot.

ascites: accumulation of fluid in the abdominal cavity.

atony: lack of energy.

Aurantiaceae: the order of trees bearing oranges, lemons, etc.

azulene: a non-aromatic hydrocarbon, usually blue, associated with sesquiterpenes (q.v.).

B

bacteriostatic: (agent) inhibiting the growth of bacteria.

bechic: (medicine) tending to cure or relieve coughing.

bedeguar: a mosslike growth on a rose-bush produced by an insect.

benzoin: a natural resin obtained from a Javanese tree; the chief constituent of friar's balsam.

bergaptene: a constituent of oil of lime.

biocatalyst: an enzyme; a substance which has a biological effect in small quantities, e.g., a vitamin.

bornyl: a radical derived from borneol.

bornyl acetate: a borneol-derived salt of acetic acid.

bornyl-isovalerianate: a borneol-derived salt of valer(ian)ic acid (q.v.).

burnet: a plant with brown flowers.

butyrate: a salt of butyric acid.

butyric aldehyde: a colourless volatile fluid derived from butter.

C

cadinene: a sesquiterpene (*q.v.*), a constituent of the essential oils of juniper and cedar.

camphene: a terpene (*q.v.*) hydrocarbon occurring in various essential oils.

caproic aldehyde: a colourless volatile fluid obtained from butter.

carcinomatosis: cancer spread throughout the body.

cardamom: an aromatic spice obtained from the seed-capsules of tropical plants of the ginger family.

cardiovascular erethism: abnormal irritability of the heart and the blood vessels.

carene: a group of terpenes (*q.v.*) found in essential oils.

carline: a genus of plants resembling the thistle.

carotene: an orange or red substance formed in carrots, etc., and acting as a source of vitamin A.

carvacrol: a compound substance extracted from camphor and origan (*q.v.*).

carveol: a constituent of essential oils of the Labiatae (*q.v.*).

carvone: a colourless liquid, the principal constituent found in oils of caraway, cumin, and dill.

caryophyllene: a mixture of sesquiterpenes (*q.v.*) forming the chief constituents of oil of cloves.

chamazulene: a blue hydrocarbon from oil of chamomile.

cheese-rennet: herbaceous plant also known as (Our)Lady's bedstraw.

Chenopodiaceae: plants of the goosefoot family.

Chenopodin: a bitter principle from *Chenopodium album*.

cholagogic: favouring the removal of bile.

cholagogue: medicine which helps to remove bile.

choline: an alcohol found in bile.

cineol: eucalyptol, a disinfectant smelling of camphor.

cinnamic acid: an aromatic acid.

citral: a terpene (q.v.) occurring in oil of lemon, orange, and lemon-grass.

citronella: a fragrant grass.

citronellal: the main constituent of oil of citronella and lemon-grass.

colibacillosis: disease caused by colon bacilli.

Compositae: order of plants with a single flower-head composed of many flowers.

coriandrol: linalool (q.v.).

coumarin: aromatic crystalline substance found in Tonka-bean seeds.

curcuma: tuberous plants yielding curry-powder.

curcumin: colouring matter of turmeric (q.v.).

cymene: a colourless liquid constituent of the oils of eucalyptus, cumin, and thyme.

cymol: a substance resembling carvacrol (q.v.) and thymol (q.v.).

D

d-borneol: one of the naturally-occurring forms of borneol (Borneo camphor).

d-camphene: a camphor-like terpene (q.v.) hydrocarbon, one of the modifications of camphene (q.v.).

deterpenise: remove the terpenes (q.v.) from.

deterpenisation: process of removing terpenes (q.v.).

dextrorotatory: rotating the plane of polarisation of light in a clockwise direction.

diaphoretic: (medicine) promoting sweating.

dihydrocarvone: a colourless liquid related to carvone (q.v.).

dipentene: a terpene (q.v.) chemically related to limonenes (q.v.).

dittany: a medicinal herb (Dictamnus albus).

diuretic: (medicine) promoting secretion of urine.

d-pinene: a type of pinene (*q.v.*).

d-sylvestrene: a modification of sylvestrene, the chief constituent of Russian and Swedish turpentine.

dysidrosis: abnormal sweat production.

E

ecchymoses: pl.of ecchymosis, escape of blood into tissues.

electuaries: pl.of electuary, a mixture of medicines with a sweet substance.

emmenagogic: inducing menstruation.

emmenagogue: medicine that induces menstruation.

empyreumatic: any odorous substance derived by distillation from vegetable or animal matter.

epigastrium: pit of the stomach.

Ericaceae: plants of the heather family.

erythrocentaurin: the red colouring matter of *Erythraea centaurium* (common centaury).

estragole: an ether of anise odour in tarragon oil.

eugenol: the chief constituent of oil of cloves and cinnamon-leaf oil, used for manufacturing vanillin (*q.v.*).

Evian: a brand of still mineral water popular in France.

F

farnesol: oil of cassia, a form of cinnamon.

flavones: yellow pigments occurring widely in plants.

flavonic: referring to flavones (*q.v.*).

furanocoumarin: a type of coumarin (*q.v.*).

furfurol: a liquid obtained from bran.

G

Gentianaceae: plants of the gentian family.

gentianaceous: referring to the plants of the gentian family.

gentiopicrin: a glucoside (*q.v.*) from gentian.

Geraniaceae: plants of the geranium family.

geraniol: a terpene (*q.v.*) alcohol forming a constituent of many esters or acid derivatives.

geranyl: the radical of geraniol (*q.v.*).

gingerin: a combination of resins and essential oils obtained from ginger.

gingerol: an essential oil from ginger.

glucides: a group term for carbohydrates and glucosides (*q.v.*).

glucoside: a vegetable compound yielding glucose.

gomenol: essence of niaouli.

Gramineae: plants of the grass family.

H

haematuria: presence of blood in urine.

haemoptysis: coughing up of blood.

haemostatic: arresting bleeding.

herniarin: a substance found in *Herniaria glabra* (rupture wort).

hetero-: combining form signifying other, different.

hydroxy-: combining form of hydroxyl, chemical radical containing hydrogen and oxygen, e.g., hydroxycitronellal, hydroxycoumarin.

hypercholesterolaemia: excessive, cholesterol in the blood.

I

icterus: jaundice.

imperatorin: a crystalline principle derived from masterwort.

indol(e): a crystalline substance related to indigo.

inulin: a carbohydrate derived from elecampane roots.

irone: the fragrant principle of violets.

isoborneol: a highly volatile alcohol.

isomer: one of two or more substances with the same atoms differently arranged and hence having different properties.

K

ketone: one of a class of organic compounds.

ketonic turmerone: a pungent sesquiterpene (q.v.) constituent of curcuma (q.v.).

L

Labiatae: an order of plants with lipped flowers, four-cornered stems, and opposite branches.

lactone: a compound produced by intramolecular condensation of an acid containing oxygen with the elimination of water.

laevorotatory: rotating the plane of polarisiation of light in an anticlockwise direction.

Lauraceae: the laurel family of aromatic shrubs and trees.

leditannic acid: a tannin formed from the Ledum genus of plants.

leuco-anthocyanidins: substances occurring in the red, blue, and purple colourings of flowers.

Liliaceae: plants of the lily family.

limonenes: compounds present in the oils of orange-peel and fir-cones.

linalool: a terpine (q.v.) of bergamot-like odour occurring in oil of coriander.

linalyl: chemical radical from linalool (q.v.).

lipids: fats found in living tissue.

l-pinene: a type of pinene (q.v.).

lupus: an ulcerous disease of the skin.

lymphatism: enlargement of the lymphatic tissue throughout the body.

M

Magnoliaceae: the magnolia family.

menthone: a dextrorotatory (q.v.) colourless liquid.

methyl anthranilate: colourless crystals soluble in alcohol, a salt of anthranilic acid.

methylchavicol: estragole (q.v.).

methyl salicylate: the main constituent of oil of
    wintergreen.
metritis: inflammation of the womb.
multivalent: having a valency of 3 or more.
myricetrin: a glucoside (q.v.) resembling quercitrin
    (q.v.).
Myristicaceae: plants of the nutmeg family.
myristic acid: a crystalline solid found in milk and
    vegetable oils.
myristicin: a yellow liquid derivative of oil of
    nutmeg.
Myrtaceae: the myrtle family of plants.

N

nerol: an alcohol derived from neroli (q.v.) oil.
neroli: an oil distilled from orange flowers.
neurovegetative dystonia: lack of tonicity of the
    autonomous nervous system.
nicotinamide: a vitamin of the B-complex, vitamin
    PP.
nigelline: an alkaloid found in the seeds of *Nigella
    sativa*.

O

ocimene: a terpene (q.v.) derived from the oil of
    sweet basil.
oligo-: combining form signifying few, little, slight.
oliguria: excessively low excretion of urine.
origan: marjoram.
origanol: sabinene (q.v.).
oxyures: parasitic worms.

P

parenchyma: tissue of cells of about equal length
    and breadth placed side by side.
pericarp: the wall of a fruit.
phellandrene: a terpene (q.v.) with two forms.
phellandrenic: of phellandrene (q.v.).

phenylacetic ester: a derivative of phenylacetic acid.

phenylethyl: a chemical radical.

phytotherapy: the use of plants for healing purposes.

pinenes: the chief constituents of oil of turpentine, eucalyptus, juniper, etc.

pinocamphone: a ketone (*q.v.*) found in oil of hyssop.

Q

quanta: pl.of quantum, a minimum amount of some entity such that all other amounts of that entity occurring in nature are multiples of it.

quercetin: a yellow dye.

quercitrin: a substance found in oak bark, tea leaves, hops, and horse-chestnut.

R

Ranunculaceae: plants of the buttercup family.

rhizome: an underground stem producing both roots and shoots.

Rosaceae: plants of the rose family.

Rutaceae: plants of the rue family.

S

sabinene: a terpene (*q.v.*) derivative from oil of marjoram.

sabinol: an alcohol derived from the oil of *Juniperus Sabina* (savine oil).

safrole: a colourless oil found in sassafras oil.

salviol: thujone (*q.v.*).

Santalaceae: trees of the sandalwood family.

santalol: terpenes (*q.v.*) from sandalwood.

santolina: a fragrant evergreen shrub with yellow flowers, also called lavender cotton.

saponins: vegetable compounds that act as emulsifiers of oils.

sclareol: the principal constituent of oil of sage.

sesquiterpenes: a group of terpene (*q.v.*) derivatives.

sinus arrhythmia: abnormal pulse.

stomatitis: inflammation of the mucous membrane of the mouth.

Syngenesia: Compositae (*q.v.*).

T

tachycardia: abnormally fast heartbeat.

taenia: tapeworm.

terebenthene: turpentine.

teresantalic alcohols: alcohols found in oil of sandalwood.

terpenes: compounds of five types occurring in plants.

terpineol: a colourless crystalline substance used extensively in perfumery.

thujone: a dextrorotatory (*q.v.*) colourless liquid obtained from the essential oils of Thuja and Salvia.

thymol: an aromatic constituent of oil of thyme, used as an antiseptic and related to carvacrol (*q.v.*)

Tiliaceae: plants belonging to the lime family.

tormentil: a medicinal herb with yellow flowers.

triterpene: one of the five types of terpenes (*q.v.*).

turmeric: an aromatic plant of the ginger family.

U

umbel: flower cluster with stalks radiating from a single point.

Umbelliferae: plants of the umbel (*q.v.*)-bearing order.

V

Valerianaceae: plants of the valerian family.

valer(ian)ic acid: a fatty acid with several isomers (*q.v.*) occurring in valerian.

valer(ian)ic aldehyde: a colourless volatile fluid obtained from valer(ian)ic acid (*q.v.*).

vanillin: a crystalline compound found in vanilla
    pods, etc.
vermifugal: expelling worms.
vermifuge: medicine that expels worms.
vitexin: a pigment found in *Vitex lucens*.
vitexinerhamnoside: a glucoside (*q.v.*).
vulnerary: a remedy that heals wounds.

Y

-yl: suffix denoting a radical, e.g., allyl, bornyl,
    geranyl.
ylangol: an isomer (*q.v.*) of geraniol (*q.v.*) from
    ylang-ylang (*q.v.*) oil.
ylang-ylang: Malayan and Philippine tree with
    perfume-bearing flowers.

Z

Zingiberaceae: plants of the ginger family.
zingiberine: the chief constituent of oil of ginger.
zona: shingles.

Aromatic oils can be obtained from

Aromatic Oil Company
12 Littlegate Street
Oxford OX1 1QT (Tel. 0865 42144)

A Doctor's Guide to

HELPING YOURSELF WITH HOMOEOPATHIC REMEDIES

James H. Stephenson, M.D.

Homoeopathy treats people, not just diseases, and a practising homoeopathic doctor here shows how you can employ scores of remedies to treat effectively a wide range of ailments and illnesses, quickly and easily. Homoeopathy is a simple programme of medical applications that has already brought long-lasting relief to thousands of people. The key to its wonder-working ability is contained in specially prepared dilutions of natural substances that are safe, inexpensive and easy to obtain.

Dr Stephenson, with over twenty years of experience in homoeopathic medicine, offers you the same straightforward and helpful treatments that he has used to bring fast relief to his own patients. There are sections devoted to treating respiratory diseases; digestive tract upsets such as colitis and constipation; bone and joint diseases like arthritis; feminine ailments; nervous troubles; skin problems and heart troubles.

Two comprehensive sections at the end of the book will help you find quick relief from a wide variety of illnesses and disorders. Firstly a complete alphabetical list of homoeopathic medicines is included with a thorough outline of the ailments that can be treated by each, and secondly there is a helpful section listing dozens of symptoms along with particular medicines that Dr Stephenson recommends for a quick recovery.

HOMOEOPATHIC GREEN MEDICINE

A.C. Gordon Ross MB, ChB, MF Hom.

Plants, trees and weeds are the sources of medicines for both the orthodox doctor and the homoeopathic practitioner, but the ways in which such medicines are prepared and administered vary widely between the two schools of thought.

Whilst the orthodox approach is to extract the active principles from plants – mostly alkaloids and glycosides – to refine and synthesize them and ultimately to prescribe them in high dosages, the homoeopathic approach is more in keeping with nature in that the whole of the plant is used in the preparation of the high dilution tinctures that constitute the homoeopath's armoury of remedies.

In this book a homoeopathic practitioner of many years experience examines the sources of what is known as 'green medicine' and, in comparing the two approaches, makes a plea for a closer liaison between allopaths – orthodox doctors – and homoeopaths. There is certainly a need for prejudices to be cast aside, and for a more open-minded approach to the efficacy of homoeopathic medicines.

EMERGENCY HOMOEOPATHIC FIRST-AID

Paul Chavanon, M.D.
and
René Levannier, M.D.

Homoeopathy alone allows the sick to be given what, above all, they ask for: remedies which are effective yet harmless. The object of this book is to provide doctors, not fully conversant with homoeopathic remedies, and the layman with no medical training at all, with a quick-reference guide to first-aid treatments for use in an emergency.

This is very important, for the promptness with which such treatment is given has a direct bearing on the speed of recovery. The suggested remedies are those found to be the most commonly effective in the long experience of the authors, the late Dr Paul Chavanon, who was laureate of the Faculty of Medicine of Paris and of the Société d'Homoeothérapie de France, and his colleague, Dr René Levannier.

In the case of the layman, the book is not supposed to be a substitute for calling the doctor, but it will enable him to take the correct action before the doctor arrives. It is a book that no household should be without. The ailments are arranged alphabetically, and remedies are given for each along with details of dosage and frequency.

HOMOEOPATHIC PRACTICE IN 30 REMEDIES

Dr E.A. Maury

The full homoeopathic clinical repertory, with its vast array of often contradictory symptoms, is very confusing for the layman. Appreciating this fact, Dr Maury has chosen thirty remedies from those which occur most frequently in homoeopathic prescriptions. Whether used by itself, or in association with one of the other twenty-nine, each remedy is designed for treating common ailments or for providing first-aid treatment while awaiting the doctor's arrival.

Successful treatment depends on the gift of observation, for every homoeopathic prescription is based on a parallel between the symptoms of the illness being treated and their medicinal correlation. As the same symptoms are frequently repeated, especially in the course of acute illnesses, the same remedies will be repeatedly indicated, and therefore these thirty prophylactics cover the bulk of the symptoms observed in the patient being treated.

Barbican Bus Special

The Barbican's answer to getting home . . .

The Barbican Bus will leave the Centre approximately 15 minutes after the matinée performances in the Hall and in the Theatre on 26, 27 December and 2 January.

The coach will set down at Charing Cross, Waterloo and Victoria Main Line Stations.

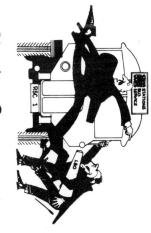

The journey time is approximately 25 minutes

Flat Fare 70p

Coach departs from Level 3 roadway

Tickets are available from the Level 3 Cloakroom counter

Angelica   Orange
Caraway   Peppermin
Carrot, wild.   Rose
Chamomiles   Rosemary
Cinnamon
Cyprus.
Eucalyptus
Ginger
Hawthorn
Lemon
Lime Blossom
Melissa
Nutmeg

Howard Blake
Sally Cavender